Abdominal Hernia Surgery - Practice, Evidence and Advances

Edited by Raimundas Lunevicius

Published in London, United Kingdom

Abdominal Hernia Surgery - Practice, Evidence and Advances
http://dx.doi.org/10.5772/intechopen.1003448
Edited by Raimundas Lunevicius

Contributors
Adam Daniel Gerrard, August Schaeffer, Hany Mohammed El-Hadi Shoukat Mohammed, Mehmet Berksun Tutan, Nazrah Shaikh, Neeraj Saxena, Raimundas Lunevicius, Rajesh Shrivastava, Richard Lu, Svetlana Doris Brincat

First published in London, United Kingdom, 2025 by IntechOpen
IntechOpen is the global imprint of INTECHOPEN LIMITED, registered in England and Wales, registration number: 11086078, 167-169 Great Portland Street, London, W1W 5PF, United Kingdom

For EU product safety concerns: IN TECH d.o.o., Prolaz Marije Krucifikse Kozulić 3, 51000 Rijeka, Croatia, info@intechopen.com or visit our website at intechopen.com.

British Library Cataloguing-in-Publication Data
A catalogue record for this book is available from the British Library

Abdominal Hernia Surgery - Practice, Evidence and Advances
Edited by Raimundas Lunevicius
p. cm.
Print ISBN 978-0-85014-799-5
Online ISBN 978-0-85014-798-8
eBook (PDF) ISBN 978-0-85014-800-8

Meet the editor

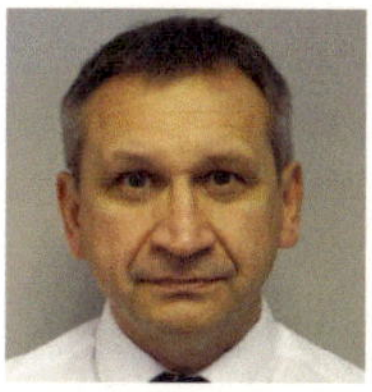

Raimundas Lunevicius, MD, Ph.D., DSc, FRCS, Professor (LT), is a Consultant in Emergency General and Trauma Surgery at Liverpool University Hospitals NHS FT, UK, with extensive experience in biliary, gastrointestinal, abdominal wall, visceral trauma surgery, research, clinical audits, education, supervision, medical appraisal, academic editing, and review. He completed three fellowship programs: Monbushou (Nagoya University & Aichi Cancer Centre, Japan, 1998–2000), Fulbright–Humphrey (Johns Hopkins University, Bloomberg School of Public Health, US, 2008–2009), and King's College Hospital (2010–2012). His publications (h-index 76) include 254 refereed articles (PubMed 161), three monographs, three book chapters, and two edited books (by 30–12–2024). He is the Editor-in-Chief of 'Emergency Care and Medicine' (MDPI, Switzerland) and a senior GBD Network collaborator.

Contents

Preface

On 1 March 2023, the '*International Journal of Surgery*' published a paper on the temporal trends in the prevalence and incidence of inguinal, femoral, umbilical, diaphragmatic, other abdominal, and unspecified abdominal hernias using the 2019 Global Burden of Disease (GBD) Study data (https://pubmed.ncbi.nlm.nih.gov/37093073/). A total of 32.5 million (95% uncertainty interval 27.7–37.8) prevalent and 13.0 million (95% uncertainty interval 10.7–15.5) incident cases of hernias were estimated globally in 2019. However, the actual prevalence and incidence of abdominal hernia is much higher, as the GBD world standard population is younger than the European, British, or US standard populations or the populations of individual countries with high sociodemographic indexes.

Approximately 75% of all abdominal wall hernias are inguinal. Although approximately 20 million individuals undergo inguinal hernia repair annually worldwide (1 million in the US), this estimate is inaccurate. Furthermore, according to the data published in the aforementioned article, an unmet need exists for abdominal wall surgery worldwide, particularly in India, the People's Republic of China, Brazil, and Central Sub-Saharan Africa. Primary midline ventral, incisional, recurrent, and parastomal hernia management is challenging within the nosological structure of the unmet need for abdominal wall hernia surgeries, and it requires constant theoretical, educational, and practical attention. Thus, the author of this preface accepted the offer to edit the open-access book project.

An invitation to contribute to this project, with six broad topics and 24 specific keywords, was circulated through social channels, including the global social hernia collaborative network. More than 30 book-chapter proposals were received, and less than 10 full-text chapters reached the editor's panel. Seven manuscripts were accepted for publication after several internal and external reviews. These manuscripts comprise this seven-chapter book for a global audience of general surgeons and allied subspecialties. The book intends to provide readers with a comprehensive overview of the current ventral hernia management and post-herniorrhaphy pain. A conceptual chapter on the open abdomen was necessary.

The first chapter, 'Laparoscopic Ventral Hernia Repair: Defect Closure Techniques', overviews the surgical anatomy of the abdominal wall, current classifications of hernia, and its repair principles. It explicitly details the ventral hernia defect extracorporeal and intracorporeal closure techniques and intraperitoneal onlay mesh placement (IPOM-Plus). Dr. Neeraj Saxena (ESIC Medical College and Hospital, Faridabad, India) emphasises that extracorporeal closure of the ventral abdominal hernia defect (component 'Plus'), following which an intraperitoneal onlay mesh is placed to cover the fascial suture (component 'IPOM'), is an innovative technique in laparoscopic ventral (including incisional) hernia surgery; it is more efficacious than historic IPOM (intraperitoneal bridging to achieve complete coverage of fascial defect using a mesh) in terms of reducing operative time, postoperative pain, seroma formation, superficial infection at the surgical site, and, therefore, hospital stay duration.

Chapter 2, 'Understanding the Neurovascular Bundle in Ventral Hernia Repair', by Dr. Rajesh Shrivastava and Dr. Nazrah Shaikh (Vedanta Institute of Medical Sciences, Shreeji Hospital, Maharashtra; Sir H. N. Reliance Foundation Hospital, Mumbai, India), comprehensively describes and illustrates the topographical anatomy of the abdominal wall. As the chapter title clearly states, its content emphasises the neurovascular bundle of the abdominal wall that plays a pivotal role in ventral hernia repairs and abdominal wall reconstructions using posterior approaches. Ten individual and compositional figures undoubtedly enhance the value of this chapter.

Chapter 3, 'Enhanced-View Totally Extraperitoneal Approach to Retrorectus Ventral Hernia Repair', by Dr. August Schaeffer and Dr. Richard Lu (University of Texas, Galveston, USA) can be described in short as 'Read, See, Plan, and Do'. It provides a precise description and eight image illustrations to potential endoscopic or robot-assisted surgery followers, provided that their surgical skills are satisfactory, exemplary, or excellent. Postoperative instructions and the range of potential site-specific complications following this novel surgical technique are also described.

Chapter 4, 'Parastomal Hernia: From Definitions and Management to Prevention', by Dr. Adam Daniel Gerrard and Dr. Raimundas Lunevicius (Liverpool University Hospitals NHS Foundation Trust, Aintree Hospital, UK), focuses on one nosological unit according to The International Statistical Classification of Diseases and Health-Related Problems (ICD-10), graded as VHWG-3 (contaminated) by both the original and modified Ventral Hernia Working Group classifications. This chapter overviews the relevant subtopics methodologically and, in a tabular form, summarises the recommendations for parastomal hernia management made by the European Hernia Society and the American Society of Colon and Rectal Surgery. The main differences between the two guidelines are highlighted.

Chapter 5, titled 'Post-Herniorrhaphy Pain: A Frequent Complication in a Common Procedure', by Dr. Mehmet Berksun Tutan (Alaca State Hospital, Çorum, Turkey), is a state-of-the-art narrative review for general surgeons based on 55 reference sources. The sixth section of this chapter, Prevention, is paramount for practitioners performing open inguinal hernia repair. Prophylactic ilioinguinal or iliohypogastric neurectomy should be considered when a nerve is suspected of being injured or at high risk of irritation due to mesh placement. An evidence-based message is provided: there is a significant reduction in chronic pain among patients undergoing prophylactic ilioinguinal or iliohypogastric neurectomy during open inguinal hernia repair without an increase in sensory deficits or surgical complications.

Chapter 6, 'Post-Herniorrhaphy Pain', by Dr. Hany Mohammed El-Hadi Shoukat Mohammed (Cairo University, Egypt), is another review, similar to the title but different in content. The emphasis on physical examinations and description of sensory and motor impairment in inguinal neuropathies, pain assessment tools, pain distribution on patients' skin mapping tests, differential diagnosis, chronic post-inguinal herniorrhaphy pain diagnostic algorithm, and management algorithm for post-herniorrhaphy groin pain makes this chapter extraordinarily valuable for practitioners.

Finally, Chapter 7, 'The Open Abdomen: A Comprehensive Narrative Review of the Life-Threatening Condition for 2024', by Dr. Svetlana Doris Brincat (Department of Surgery, Mater Dei Hospital, Malta) and Dr. Raimundas Lunevicius (Liverpool, UK), is a detailed overview of an uncommon condition wherein the key layer of the abdominal wall—musculofascial—was not closed during an abdominal surgical procedure and, therefore, left exposed to the atmosphere in one or another way by a medical intention and plan. The chapter includes tables and figures to detail the classification of temporary and definitive abdominal closure methods and illustrate surgical outcomes.

I am grateful to all authors for their excellent contributions to this project. I would also like to thank the IntechOpen staff, especially Ms. Marica Novakovic, the Publishing Process Manager, and Ms. Lucija Tomicic-Dromgool, the Senior Commissioning Editor.

Raimundas Lunevicius
Department of General Emergency and Trauma Surgery,
Liverpool University Hospitals NHS Foundation Trust,
Liverpool, UK

Chapter 1

Laparoscopic Ventral Hernia Repair: Defect Closure Techniques

Neeraj Saxena

Abstract

During laparoscopic ventral abdominal hernia repair (LVHR), defect closure utilizing extracorporeal suturing for closure of defect is compared with intracorporeal suturing. It is effective and easier with lesser complications like bowel injury, infection, and recurrence. It is done using a spinal needle and a prolene suture or a special suture grasper. It does not require much experience and training to perform this procedure. The results are excellent, reproducible, and suitable for all patients with ventral abdominal hernia. Extracorporeal closure of the ventral abdominal hernia defect in LVHR is an innovative technique to close the hernia defect following which intraperitoneal onlay mesh (IPOM-Plus) is placed to cover the defect so as to reduce chances of recurrence.

Keywords: ventral hernia, incisional hernia, extracorporeal, intracorporeal, IPOM plus, laparoscopic

1. Introduction

Ventral hernia is a prevalent surgical condition that can occur in individuals of both genders and age groups. A ventral hernia is characterized by the bulging of tissue through the fascia of the anterior abdominal wall.

2. Classification

The classification of defects is by

a. Either spontaneous or acquired, or by their location on the abdominal wall or

b. According to European Hernia Society (EHS) Classification.

Epigastric hernias arise in the midline spanning from the xiphoid process above to the umbilicus below, whereas umbilical hernias exclusively develop through the umbilicus. *Spigelian hernia* occurs in the anterior abdominal wall, in close proximity to linea semilunaris. *Hypogastric hernias* are infrequent hernias in the midline below the umbilicus that develop spontaneously.

Incisional hernias are acquired hernias following surgical incisions.

Diastasis recti, though not an actual hernia, can manifest as a bulge in the midline inbetween the two recti because of stretching of linea alba.

Of all the abdominal wall hernias, umbilical and epigastric hernias constitute 10%, whereas 15–20 percent are categorized as incisional hernias [1]. Women experience incisional hernias twice as frequently as men do.

Usually, late diastasis of the fascial planes at the incisional site or failure of fascias to heal are the causes of *incisional hernia*. Contributing factors are inadequate healing of previous incision site, excessive tension, and surgical site infection. According to Jaykar et al., the incidence in patients with surgical wound infection can rise to 46% [2]. Following abdominal surgery, incisional hernias are frequent and can disrupt the functioning of the vascular, respiratory, and other organ systems.

Protrusion of abdominal contents from the cavity in large hernias results in loss of abdominal domain. The abdominal wall loses its natural rigidity as a result, and the muscles frequently retract. Following surgical repair, reintroducing the contents of the hernia sac back into the abdominal cavity could potentially impede blood circulation or respiratory function. Domain loss is defined by the Tanaka Index (hernia sac volume more than 25% of the peritoneal volume) or by the Sabbagh method which takes hernia sac volume to be more than 20% of the total peritoneal volume.

The majority of *umbilical hernias* are present at birth and generally resolve on their own by the age of 2 years. If they persist beyond the age of 5 years, surgical correction is necessary. Adult umbilical hernias are more frequent in women and are typically acquired. During surgery, the sac is separated from the fascia and the umbilicus, and the defect is closed primarily without mesh if it is small (< 3 cm). Larger defects are sutured with prosthetic mesh overlay.

Men are more prone to have *epigastric hernias*, which can be observed in the midline from the xiphoid process to the umbilicus. The presence of small defects leads to a disproportionate amount of pain due to the entrapment of preperitoneal fat. The treatment is to excise the trapped preperitoneal tissue and the subsequent closure of the defect in the fascia.

European Hernia Society or the EHS has classified [3] ventral hernias into midline and lateral hernias. The classification defines 5 M zones and 4 L zones:

1. M1: Subxiphoidal (from the xiphoid process till 3 cm caudally)

2. M2: Epigastric (from 3 cm below the xiphoid process till 3 cm above the umbilicus)

3. M3: Umbilical (from 3 cm above till 3 cm below the umbilicus)

4. M4: Infraumbilical (from 3 cm below the umbilicus till 3 cm above the pubis)

5. M5: Suprapubic (from pubic bone till 3 cm cranially).

The four L zones on each side are defined as:

1. L1: Subcostal (between the costal margin and a horizontal line 3 cm above the umbilicus)

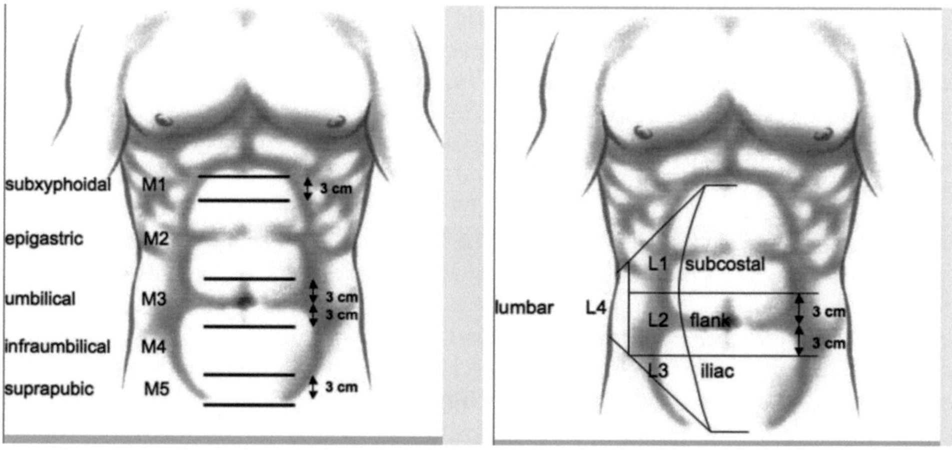

Figure 1.
EHS classification.

2. L2: Flank (lateral to the rectal sheath in the area 3 cm above and below the umbilicus)

3. L3: Iliac (between a horizontal line 3 cm below the umbilicus and the inguinal region)

4. L4: Lumbar (latero-dorsal of the anterior axillary line).

Hernias extending across two or more M zones are categorized by assigning them to the M zone which is typically regarded as challenging or hernia representative. The succession of significance for these locations is as follows: first, M1 (subxiphoid) & M5 (suprapubic), then M3 (umbilical), and finally M2 (epigastric) and M4 (infraumbilical).

Therefore, a hernia extending from M1 over M2 to M3 (that is from subxiphoidal to the umbilicus) is to be classified as M1 (that is as a subxiphoidal hernia). A hernia extending from M2 over M3 to M4 (that is from epigastric to infraumbilical) is to be classified as M3 (that is as an umbilical hernia) (**Figure 1**) [3].

Defect size is classified as W1 $<$ 4 cm; W2 $\geq$ 4–10 cm; W3 $\geq$ 10 cm.

3. Risk factors

Risk factors for ventral hernia are obesity, history of previous abdominal surgery, continuous strain on abdominal wall, infection at surgical incision site, diabetes, steroids use, pregnancy, etc. If the ventral hernia becomes irreducible, obstructed, or strangulated, surgical intervention is necessary.

Patient-related risk factors related to the formation of ventral hernias include emphysema, prostatism, sleep apnea, advanced age, obesity, as well as male sex. Wound infection predisposes to hernia formation.

The abdominal wall has enough strength to endure increased pressure in the abdomen as well as to effectively limit the protrusion of internal contents. Origin of herniation is a result of elevated pressure caused by constipation, symptoms related to the prostate, obesity, and excessive coughing in respiratory ailments.

Recent data suggests a significant association between the surgical technique used for closing a midline laparotomy and the occurrence of incisional hernias. Most surgeons frequently use 1 cm bites and 1 cm advancement suturing to close the laparotomy. It is suggested that a suture to wound length ratio of 4:1 is a better method to close the midline laparotomy, and it results in a much lesser incidence of incisional hernias [4].

Patients with hernia have an inherited imbalance in various types of collagen and are, therefore, classified as a collagen disorder. Collagen type I is typically found in mature scars or fascial tissues, whereas in the initial stages of wound healing, collagen type III predominates which has fewer cross-links, making it mechanically weaker and less stable.

The study conducted by Peeters E, DeHertogh G, and Junge K in 2014 analyzed the ratio of collagen type I to collagen type III in individuals with primary inguinal hernia, recurrent inguinal hernia, primary incisional hernia, and recurrent incisional hernia [5]. The cases demonstrated a substantial increase in the proportion of collagen III found within the skin and anterior rectus sheath fascia resulting in a decrease in the ratio of collagen type I to type III in incisional and recurrent inguinal hernia patients than that of primary inguinal hernia patients.

Hernia is a frequent occurrence during pregnancy because the ligaments become more relaxed. It is also prevalent in elderly individuals as a result of the weakening of muscles and fibrous tissue due to degenerative changes.

4. Components of ventral hernia

Ventral hernia has two essential components, an abnormality in the wall causing a defect in it along with contents (tissue) that has been displaced outside the abdominal cavity. A small defect within the rigid walls traps the displaced contents and restricts their movement between compartments, which can lead to complications.

5. Surgical anatomy

The *anterior abdominal wall* consists of three layers of muscles, the fascicles in each layer are oriented obliquely at varying angles to form a robust covering that encloses the contents of the abdomen. In the midline, the aponeuroses of these muscles are inserted within the linea alba, a central structure that connects the two sides of the wall of abdomen.

The *external oblique* is the lateral abdominal wall's superficially located muscle. The internal oblique muscle is situated beneath the external oblique muscle and the transversus abdominis muscle situated beneath the internal oblique forms the third layer. The fibers of the external oblique muscle run in a downward and inward direction. The fibers of the *internal oblique* muscle are located beneath the external oblique muscle and directed perpendicular to it. The fibers of the *transversus abdominis* muscle run horizontally. The three lateral muscles become aponeurotic adjacent to the Recti, which continue towards midline to form the anterior as well as posterior layers of the rectus sheath. The two anterior rectus sheaths proceed to join in the midline to form the tendinous *linea alba*. The rectus abdominis muscles are located on either side of the linea alba. Their fibers are aligned vertically in a longitudinal manner and extend from xiphoid process to pubic symphysis. The posterior layer of the rectus sheath is located beneath each rectus muscle and also contributes towards the formation of the linea alba.

The external oblique aponeurosis continues inward to constitute the anterior layer of the sheath of the rectus. The *arcuate line*, a key anatomical landmark in hernia repairs, is found on the posterior aspect of the anterior abdominal wall, located around 3–6 cm beneath the umbilicus.

The two laminae of the aponeurosis of the internal oblique muscle form the front and back coverings of the rectus abdominis muscle above the arcuate line. *Above* the arcuate line, posterior sheath is formed by the posterior lamina of the internal oblique and the transversus abdominis. The posterior rectus sheath is absent *below* the arcuate line and consists of only the transversalis fascia and the peritoneum.

The nerve supply to the abdominal wall is through intercostal nerves and 1st and 2nd lumbar nerves. These nerves supplying the lateral abdominal muscles, the rectus muscle, and the overlying skin travel specifically in the space between the internal oblique muscles and transversus abdominis, and just medial to the linea semilunaris they pierce the posterior rectus sheath to supply the rectus muscle. During hernia repair surgery by transversus abdominis release (TAR), it is important to preserve these nerves supplying the rectus muscle.

The blood supply to the abdominal wall is by lumbar arteries, deep circumflex iliac artery, and lower three or four intercostal arteries. The blood supply to the rectus muscle is derived from the superior and inferior epigastric arteries. These are branches of internal mammary artery and external iliac artery, respectively. In addition the lower intercostal arteries also contribute. An anastomosis forms between the superior and inferior epigastric arteries near the umbilicus. Skin flap necrosis is a potential complication if the anastomotic vessels around the umbilicus are damaged during surgery.

6. The pre-peritoneal fat

Complex abdominal wall repair during abdominal wall reconstruction requires extended retromuscular dissection. It is essential to comprehend the anatomy of the peritoneal layer and abdominal wall muscles, specifically the preperitoneal fat. The preperitoneal fat displays a morphology resembling a trident.

This preperitoneal fat located beneath the linea alba takes on a rhomboid shape as it extends upwards in the midline towards the epigastric region.

Below the arcuate line, the fat located in the midline preperitoneal area extends downwards towards the Retzius space.

Bogros space, also known as the retroinguinal space, is located laterally, and it communicates with the Retzius space in the midline. This space also anatomically connects the base of the trident-shaped structure to the paracolic gutters, the Toldt's fascia as well as pararenal fats which constitute the lateral branches of the trident.

Understanding the anatomy of the preperitoneal fatty trident [6] is essential for carrying out different types of hernia surgeries, including simple ventral hernia repair and more intricate procedures like preperitoneal ventral repair or posterior component separation techniques. The surgeon can extend the preperitoneal dissection inbetween the peritoneum and muscle layers in these consistent pathways.

7. Evaluation of ventral hernias

The *evaluation of abdominalwall hernia* necessitates thorough physical examination along with imaging. Similar to the inguinal region, the evaluation of the anterior abdominal wall involves assessing patients in standing as well as supine positions. Additionally, performing actions such as coughing, raising the head or legs, or using a Valsalva maneuver can be helpful in identifying and determining the size as well as location of a hernia.

The utilization of advanced imaging techniques, such as the CT scan, is becoming increasingly advantageous in assessing the site, size, extent of the hernia, the strength of tissues around the hernia defect, and loss of domain. It is also valuable in detection of infrequent hernias affecting the wall of abdominal.

8. Repair techniques

Primary repair of ventral hernias is possible when defect is of a small size (less than 2–3 cm in diameter), and there is healthy surrounding tissue. Primary closure of larger defects has a significantly higher likelihood of recurrence of hernia and therefore requires prosthetic mesh, the use of which results in a substantial decline in rates of recurrence, dropping from 63 to 32.6% [7]. The primary objective of prosthetic mesh is to promote adequate tissue ingrowth, primarily consisting of type 1 collagen, in order to provide the necessary mechanical strength to prevent the recurrence of the hernia. The presence of mesh in the body triggers an immune response, akin to a response to a foreign body, leading to the formation of fibrous tissue around the mesh.

Therefore, utilization of mesh in tension-free repair is widely acknowledged as the present day standard of excellence.

Primary repair of incisional hernias defect is possible when it is small (≤ 2–3 cm diameter) and surrounded by healthy tissue, or in instances where the hernia is evidently due to a technical error during the previous surgery, like broken suture.

Defects that are greater than 2–3 cm in diameter have substantial likelihood of recurring if they are closed primarily and are therefore repaired with a prosthesis. The rates of recurrence range from 10–50% [8] and are usually decreased by over 50% when prosthetic mesh is utilized. Prosthetic material can be used to reinforce a tissue repair by placing it as an onlay patch, inserting it between the fascial defect or positioning it amongst the planes of tissue, or placing it in a sublay retrorectus position.

9. Laparoscopic repair of ventral hernias

Laparoscopic method for repairing ventral hernias was introduced by Leblanc and Booth in 1993 [9]. This approach has been widely acknowledged to provide certain advantages like faster recovery, shorter hospital stays, reduction in wound infection, and lower recurrence rates. It is contraindicated in emergency situations such as cases of hemodynamic instability or incarcerated hernia with or without gangrenous bowel. For managing patients with a hostile abdomen, such as those with enterocutaneous fistulae, a history of open abdomen, severe abdominal injuries, or prior extensive surgeries, an open approach is recommended. The decision to use the laparoscopic approach in these cases should be guided by the skill of the surgeon alongwith the likelihood of achieving a safe intra-abdominal access.

The laparoscopic surgical method for ventral hernia repair is increasingly favored by patients and surgeons due to its less invasive nature and reduced morbidity compared to traditional surgery. The method is an advancement on the open preperitoneal sublay repair technique outlined by Rives and Stoppa as mentioned by Oprea V, Toma M et al. in their publication [10].

Laparoscopic ventral hernia repair was originally designed as an intraperitoneal *bridge repair* (inlay) at an underlay site to achieve complete coverage of fascial defect by a mesh.

In recent times, there has been a growing inclination for carrying out *primary fascial closure* bringing the fascia back together prior to placing the mesh. Supporters of primary fascial closure argue that closing the fascia can enhance the functionality of the abdominal wall, decrease the likelihood of recurrence by achieving a greater degree of fascial overlap with the mesh, and reduce the production of seromas by minimizing the dead space between the mesh and the surrounding tissues [11, 12].

Fascial defects in laparoscopic ventral hernia repair can be closed using extracorporeal and intracorporeal suturing techniques.

10. Techniques of ventral hernia defect closure

An IPOM-Plus hernia repair involves the defect closure in the fascia using either *extracorporeal or intracorporeal techniques*, utilizing continuous or interrupted non absorbable sutures.

The transfascial suture passer needle has been utilized by most surgeons for the purpose of primary fascial closure during laparoscopic IPOM-Plus hernia repair [13].

Lai Jun Han [14] in a case report in 2019 titled "A novel alternative to suture passer for closure of the fascial defect in LVHR" concluded that an IV cannula or spinal needle can be utilized as a cost-effective substitute for a transfascial suture passer needle (**Figure 2**).

This report, published in 2019, was the first to explore the use of an IV cannula as a substitute for a suture passer needle in laparoscopic IPOM repair for fascial closure. Unlike the suture passer needle, this innovative needle and suture is cheaper, readily available, and being disposable and has no risk of transmitting disease. Furthermore, due to its narrower diameter compared to a suture passer needle, it can be inserted effectively without much force. The technique is easily learnt, requires no training, and is highly replicable. The results are excellent and reproducible.

Whether the defect is bridged or closed with sutures, the subsequent surgery involves mesh placement and mesh fixation.

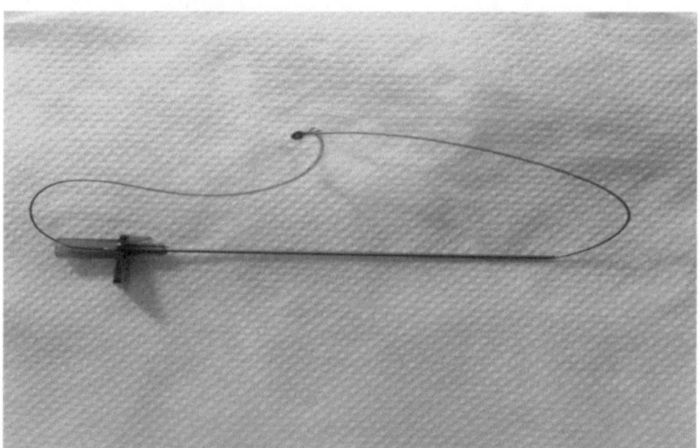

Figure 2.
Spinal needle with prolene suture: an alternative to the traditional suture passer needle.

11. Mesh placement

Surgeons have multiple choices for positioning the mesh, as even the tiniest ventral hernia can be effectively treated using mesh. The European Hernia Society defines four classic mesh planes for ventral hernia repair: onlay, inlay, sublay, and underlay (**Figure 3**):

The onlay (overlay) technique The procedure involves applying a mesh directly over the sutured defect in the anterior fascia. One notable benefit of this technique is that the mesh is positioned outside the abdominal cavity, thus preventing direct contact with the abdominal viscera. Nevertheless, there are several drawbacks associated with this procedure. Firstly, it requires an elaborate dissection of the subcutaneous tissue flaps, which significantly raises the chances of vascular and nerve injuries to the skin flap and seroma formation, infection, and flap necrosis.

In the sublay (underlay) technique, a mesh is positioned beneath the fascial components. The mesh could be positioned *retrorectus (retromuscular) space*, *preperitoneally or intraperitoneally*. This technique of placing the mesh beneath the fascia is strongly recommended. The mesh is held in place and prevented from moving or shifting by the natural forces within the cavity of abdomen due to the mesh's wide coverage.

The *intraperitoneal onlay mesh (IPOM)* technique is a specific surgical procedure in which a mesh is placed into the abdominal cavity in an onlay position from inside the abdomen, thereby covering the hernia defect.

Once the hernia opening is fully exposed, a decision must be taken as to whether a composite mesh can be placed directly over the defect as a form of bridge repair

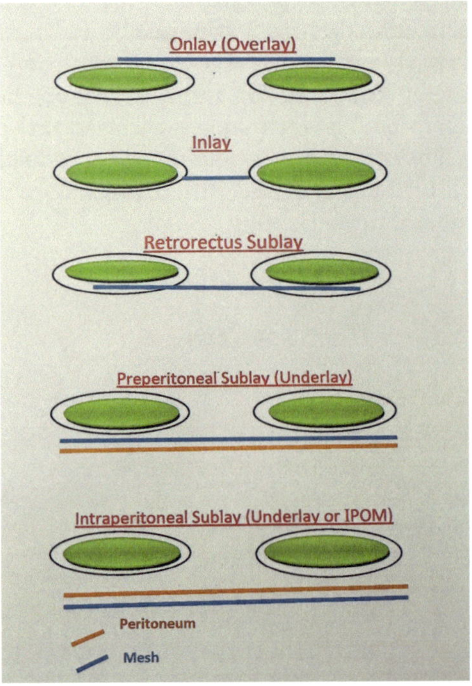

Figure 3.
Mesh positions in ventral hernia repair.

(IPOM) or whether the defect must be additionally constricted with a suture so that the synthetic mesh is better supported (IPOM-Plus technique).

12. Mesh fixation

Mesh fixation is a pivotal step in LVHR. The primary objective is to prevent mesh migration and minimize postoperative pain and recurrence. Different techniques of mesh fixation are suture, staple, or tack. Intracorporeal and transfascial suture fixation technique are used to fix the mesh by suture. Both absorbable as well as nonabsorbable tackers are utilized to fix the mesh to the abdominal wall.

After dealing with the hernia sac and its contents, mesh equipped with multiple sutures is inserted and unfolded over the abdominal wall defect. Using the suture passer needle, the visible paired strands on the mesh corners are guided out through tiny punctures in the skin of the abdominal wall and secured to the abdominal wall fascia by tying knots through these small punctures. This allows for the secure attachment of the mesh to the abdominal wall at its corners. Furthermore, the synthetic mesh is fastened internally using specialized tacks equipped with nonabsorbable titanium spirals or absorbable screws in a double crowning fashion.

13. Mesh types

Presently, the global annual usage of meshes amounts to approximately one million [15].

Meshes fall into two major categories:

1. Synthetic and

2. Biologic.

Synthetic meshes are either nondegradable or degradable.

Biologic meshes are all biodegradable.

An ideal mesh should be chemically inert, hypoallergenic, sterilizable, resistant to mechanical stress without compromising compliance, and causing minimal inflammatory response.

Mesh is also categorized according to its water angle (hydrophobic or hydrophilic), weight, pore size, and presence or absence of an antiadhesive barrier (**Tables 1–3**).

Composite meshes were created to reduce the side effects of meshes and are composed of two or more discrete components. A lot of composite meshes are what are known as "*biface implants*"—that is, they have smooth microporous interior surfaces to prevent adhesions when in contact with viscera and porous exterior surfaces that promote tissue integration. The visceral surface can contain any combination of synthetic or biological materials, degradable or nondegradable. This material could be 3 k cellulose, monocryl, omega-3, hyaluronate, titanium, polyvinylidene fluoride, polyglactin, polyglecaprone, and collagen. The external surface is typically composed of a nondegradable synthetic material [16, 17].

There is another class of composite meshes which is *not biface*; instead, it is made of a synthetic mesh that is nondegradable and coated with a transient barrier [17]. Meshes with temporary barrier coatings have a biodegradable barrier layer made of

Polypropylene	Prolene	Rigid, inert used in most woven prosthesis
	Marlex	
	Parietene	
	Surgipro	
Polyethlene terephthalate	Dacron	Elastic, hydrophilic
Expanded Polytetrafluoroethylene (ePTFE)	Goretex	Rigid, hydrophobic, low integration
	Teflon	decreases risk of adhesions

Table 1.
Synthetic non degradable meshes.

Material	Mesh	Degradation time
Polyglactin	Vicryl	1–3 months
Polyglycolic acid	Dexon	1–3 months
Polyglycolic acid/Trimethylene carbonate	Gore Bio A	6 Months
Poly 4 hydroxybutyrate	Phasix	12–18 months

Table 2.
Synthetic degradable meshes.

Allogenic Human Dermis	Alloderm(Lifecell, USA)
	Allomax (Bard Davol Inc. USA)
	Flex HD (Ethicon, USA)
Xenogenic Porcine Dermis	Permacol (Medtronic, USA)
	Collamend (Bard Davol Inc., USA)
	Strattice (Lifecell" USA)

Table 3.
Biologic degradable mesh materials.

a substance that prevents the formation of adhesions; these materials are typically hydrophilic coatings like collagen. In other words, in theory, they facilitate incorporation as well as inhibit adhesion formation during the initial phase of implantation, and once the coating degrades, they transform into a regular synthetic nondegradable mesh.

Currently available composite mesh examples include C-Qur (Atrium Medical, USA), Vypro (Ethicon, USA), Ti-mesh (Medtronic, USA) Dynamesh (FEG Textiltechnik, Germany), Parietex composite (Medtronic, USA), Proceed (Ethicon, USA), Ventralight ST (Bard Davol Inc., USA), Sepramesh (Bard Davol Inc., USA), Ultrapro (Ethicon, USA), and Composix (Bard Davol Inc., USA).

The visceral side of expanded polytetrafluoroethylene (ePTFE) composite mesh is microporous (3 micrometers), while the abdominal wall side is macroporous. A macroporous mesh without any protective covering is suitable for positioning it outside the peritoneal cavity without causing damage to the bowel. Hydrophobic macroporous polypropylene mesh permits native fibroblast ingrowth and integration into the surrounding fascia.

In 1998, the first lightweight meshes, specifically Vypro, were introduced to tackle the enduring problems associated with heavyweight polypropylene mesh.

Mesh can be classified according to its weight

1. Lightweight mesh (Less than 40 g/m^2)

2. Medium weight mesh (40–60 g/m^2)

3. Heavy weight mesh (75 g/m^2).

These lightweight meshes, which are usually made of Vicryl (Polyglactin 910) or Monocryl, offer initial handling stability. These meshes have large pores of size around 3 to 5 mm with a small surface area. They have greater elasticity and flexibility [17] as they stimulate reduced inflammatory reactions. They usually shrink less and are found to have less pain. Although there have been some improvements, complications such as recurrences, infection, and adhesion formation still persist. Therefore, a perfect mesh has not yet been discovered.

The challenges faced with synthetic materials prompted the advancement of biomaterials for the creation of implants that closely mimic physiological conditions. These biomaterials are composed of an acellular collagen matrix obtained from either porcine small intestine submucosa (known as Surgisis) or human dermis (known as Aderm). The matrix facilitates the infiltration of soft tissue into the mesh, leading to its integration into the body through a process of remodeling.

14. Outcome and postoperative complications

According to the research performed by *Suwa et al.* [18] in 2016 titled "Closure versus non-closure of fascial defects in laparoscopic ventral and incisional hernia repairs" showed that the mesh bulging, rates of recurrence, and seroma formation had been 0–7.7 percent, 0–11.4 percent, and zero percent, respectively.

Primary fascial closure has been a proven technique that can reduce the seroma formation and bulging, and also the rates of recurrence, while also improving patient contentment and QoL.

IPOM-Plus appears to be more efficacious than IPOM for the treatment of large incisional hernias, specifically in terms of mitigating mesh bulging. Research conducted by *Suwa et al.* [19] titled "Is fascial defect closure with intraperitoneal onlay mesh superior to standard intraperitoneal onlay mesh for laparoscopic repair of large incisional hernia?" the study determined that the duration of the operation had been 150 minutes for IPOM as well as 148 minutes for IPOM-Plus (P = 0.6220).

Four out of twelve IPOM patients (33%) and three out of fourteen IPOM-Plus patients (21%) experienced *early postoperative complications*, specifically seroma formation (P = 0.6652). The amount of mesh bulging had been considerably greater with IPOM compared to IPOM-Plus (50% vs. 0%; P = 0.0082). Two cases of IPOM-Plus (14%) experienced chronic pain lasting for 3 months after the operation, but this occurrence did not have statistical significance.

Patients who underwent IPOM surgery had a longer duration of hospitalization compared to patients who underwent IPOM-Plus surgery. There was only one instance of recurrence in the IPOM group, which accounted for 8% of the cases. However, this finding did not reach statistical significance. IPOM-Plus appears to be more efficacious than IPOM for the treatment of large incisional hernias, specifically in terms of mitigating mesh bulging.

In another study done in 2022 at ABVIMS & Dr. Ram Manohar Lohia Hospital, New Delhi, India, a net of 32 cases of ventral hernia underwent LVHR comparing extracorporeal suture of the defect with the intracorporeal suturing.

This study was a randomized comparative study. The patients had been allocated randomly into two groups.

1. Group 1—Extracorporeal closure of defect and

2. Group 2—Intracorporeal closure of defect.

Both groups were evaluated for several factors including operative time, seroma formation, postoperative pain, seroma formation, superficial surgical site infection, duration of hospital stay as well as early recurrence (if any) within a 3-month follow-up period.

The following variables were significantly associated ($p < 0.05$)

1. Operative time (minutes),

2. Seroma formation,

3. Pain,

4. Superficial SSI, and

5. Hospital stay.

The frequency of occurrences of these complications in the intracorporeal group was significantly greater than in the extracorporeal group.

15. Robotic ventral hernia repair

Finally, with the advent of robotic hernia repair, concerns including seroma formation pain and recurrence are reduced compared to routine laparoscopic extracorporeal or intracorporeal closure of defect along with placement of intraperitoneal onlay mesh (IPOM-Plus). This reduction in the postoperative pain is particularly notable because mesh is secured through intracorporeal suturing, eliminating the need for transfascial suture or tackers.

Schluender et al. [20] in 2003 research presented the initial application of robotic technology employing the porcine model for ventral hernia repair. Central as well as circumferential sutures were used to secure the hernia, and the results demonstrated that the robotic approach allowed for easier intracorporeal suturing and unmatched accuracy in suture placement when compared to traditional laparoscopy.

The research performed by *Schluender et al.* [20] in 2003 titled "Robot-assisted laparoscopic repair of ventral hernia with intracorporeal suturing" concluded that the transabdominal sutures with tackers utilized in LVHR may serve as the primary source of postoperative pain as well as adhesions. Alternatively, the da Vinci Robot could utilize to assist in performing intracorporeal suturing of the mesh directly to the fascial edge and also to suture the mesh's circumference to the posterior fascia. The initial results are encouraging and demonstrate a secure approach that can be adopted.

The comparative research studies examining the use of robotic-assisted laparoscopic ventral hernia repair with closure of the fascial defect, as compared to laparoscopic ventral hernia repair without fascial defect closure, revealed a lower incidence of recurrence as well as complications in the group of patients that received robotic assisted surgery. Utilizing robotic technology for ventral hernia repair delivers a distinct advantage. Robotic technology enables the performance of intricate repairs, like the pre-peritoneal placement technique with subsequent closure of the peritoneum, that can potentially eliminate the requirement for a dual mesh. From a technical standpoint, the utilization of robotic technology can simplify the process of handling and deploying mesh, thus eliminating the requirement for mesh deployment devices, trans-fascial sutures, or tackers.

16. Conclusions and recommendations

It is concluded that the technique of extracorporeal closure of fascial.

defect in LVHR has better outcomes than intracorporeal closure of fascial defect in terms.

of operative time, postoperative pain, seroma formation, superficial infection at the surgical site, and the length of hospital stay. The extracorporeal technique of hernia defect closure in LVHR is, therefore, recommended by the author.

Author details

Neeraj Saxena
ESIC Medical College and Hospital, Faridabad, Haryana State, India

*Address all correspondence to: neerajsaxena27@gmail.com

References

[1] Townsend CM, Beauchamp RD, Evers BM, Mattox KL. Sabiston Textbook of Surgery: The Biological Basis of Modern Surgical Practice. 20th ed. Philadelphia, PA: Elsevier Saunders; 2017

[2] Jaykar RD, Varudkar AS, Akamanchi AK. A clinical study of ventral hernia. International Journal of Surgery. 2017;**44**(7):2326-2329

[3] Muysoms FE, Miserez M, Berrevoet F, Campanelli G, et al. Classification of primary and abdominal wall hernias. Hernia. 2009;**13**(4):407-414

[4] Beeson S, Faulkner J, Acquista E, Hope W. Decreasing incisional hernia by teaching 4:1 suture to wound lengthratio early in surgical education. Journal of Surgical Education. 2021;**78**(6):169-e173. DOI: 10.1016/j.jsurg.2021.09.008, Epub 2021 Oct 9

[5] Peeters E, DeHertogh G, Junge K. Klinge U-skin as marker for collagen type I/III ratio in abdominal wall fascia. Hernia. 2014;**18**(4):519-525. DOI: 10.1007/s10029-013-1128-1. Epub 2013 Jun 22

[6] Garcia Urena MA, Moncluz L. Pathways of the preperitoneal plane: From the "fatty triangle" in rives to the "fatty trident" in extended retromuscular abdominal wall reconstruction. A tribute to prof. Schumpelick. Hernia. 2023;**27**(2):395-407

[7] Burger JW, Luijendijk RW, Hop WC, Halm JA, Verdaasdonk EG, Jeekel J. Long-term follow-up of a randomized controlled trial of suture versus mesh repair of incisional hernia. Annals of Surgery. 2004;**240**(4):578-583; discussion 583-5. DOI: 10.1097/01.sla.0000141193.08524.e7

[8] Malviya A, Patel A, Bhardwaj G, Bulchandani HP. Saini V.A comprehensive study on the incidence and management of incisional hernia. International Journal of Surgery. 2017;**4**:2303-2307

[9] LeBlanc KA, Booth WV, Whitaker JM, Bellanger DE. Laparoscopic incisional and ventral herniorrhaphy in 100 patients. The American Journal of Surgery. 2000;**180**(3):193-197. ISSN 0002-9610

[10] Oprea V, Toma M, Grad O, Moga D. Tips and tricks for a sound rives - Stoppa repair. Annals of Surgical Education. 2022;**3**(1):1028

[11] Aljohani E. Closure versus non-closure of hernia defect in laparoscopic ventral hernia repair with mesh: A systematic review. The Indian Journal of Surgery. 2021. DOI: 10.1007/s12262-021-03203-4

[12] Elwan AM, Eid M, et al. Comparitive study between fascial defect closure and non-closure in laparoscopic incisional and ventral repair of hernia. IJMA. 2019;**1**(1):1

[13] Lasheen AE, AbdElaal S, Alkilany M, Alnaimy T, Ibrahim A, Baiomy T, et al. Percutaneous trans-abdominal external needle for hernia defect closure in laparoscopic repair. Edorium Journal of Surgery. 2016;**5**:18-23

[14] Lai JH, Loo GH, Shuhaili MAB, Ritza KN. A novel alternative to suture passer for closure of fascial defect in laparoscopic ventral hernia repair. A case reports. International Journal of Surgery Case Reports. 2019;**60**:276-280. DOI: 10.1016/j.ijscr.2019.06.045

[15] Rastengarpour A, Cheung M, Vardhan M, Ibrahim MM, Butler CE,

Levinson H. Surgical mesh for incisional hernia repairs: Understanding mesh design. Plastic Surgery (Oakv). 2016;**24**(1):41-50

[16] Bilsel Y, Abci I. The search for ideal hernia repair; mesh materials and types. International Journal of Surgery. 2012;**10**:317-321

[17] Cevasco M, Itani KM. Ventral hernia repair with synthetic, composite, and biologic mesh: Characteristics, indications, and infection profile. Surgical Infections. 2012;**13**:209-215

[18] Suwa K, Okamoto T, Yanaga K. Closure versus non-closure of fascial defects in laparoscopic ventral and incisional hernia repairs: A review of the literature. Surgery Today. 2016;**46**(7):764-773. DOI: 10.1007/s00595-015-1219-y. Epub 2015 Jul 22

[19] Suwa K, Okamoto T, Yanaga K. Is fascial defect closure with intraperitoneal onlay mesh superior to standard intraperitoneal onlay mesh for laparoscopic repair of large incisional hernia? Asian Journal of Endoscopic Surgery. 2018;**11**(4):378-384. DOI: 10.1111/ases.12471. Epub 2018 Mar 23

[20] Schluender S, Conrad J, Divino CM, Gurland B. Robot-assisted laparoscopic repair of ventral hernia with intracorporeal suturing. Surgical Endoscopy. 2003;**17**(9):1391-1395. DOI: 10.1007/s00464-002-8795-9. Epub 2003 Jun 25

Chapter 2

Understanding the Neurovascular Bundle in Ventral Hernia Repair

Rajesh Shrivastava and Nazrah Shaikh

Abstract

A ventral hernia is an abnormal protrusion of an organ or tissue through a defect in the anterior abdominal wall. Such defects may occur spontaneously or arise due to a weakened abdominal wall musculature or due to previous surgical incisions. Despite being a common surgical condition, ventral hernias can prove to be a complex clinical entity, especially due to the myriad of techniques available for their repair. A common crucial denominator in all these procedures is the meticulous identification, handling and preservation of the neurovascular bundle. It is imperative to have a thorough understanding of the anatomy of the abdominal wall including it's fascia, musculature and neurovascular structures, in order to ensure good clinical outcomes and prevent further complications. This chapter shall explore the detailed anatomy of the neurovascular bundle, it's clinical significance and role in ventral hernia repairs and strategies to avoid damage to the neurovascular bundle and further complications.

Keywords: hernia, ventral hernia repair, neurovascular bundle, anterior abdominal wall anatomy, component separation

1. Introduction

A ventral hernia is an abnormal protrusion of an organ or tissue through a defect in the anterior abdominal wall. Such defects may occur spontaneously or arise due to a weakened abdominal wall musculature or due to previous surgical incisions. Ventral hernias can be complex entities, especially when using various novel techniques for their repair. A common crucial denominator in all these procedures is the meticulous identification, handling, and preservation of the neurovascular bundle. A comprehensive literature review was conducted by systematically searching databases such as PubMed Central and Directory of Open Access Journals to identify relevant articles. The search strategy focused on keywords like ventral hernia repair, neurovascular bundle, anterior abdominal wall anatomy, and component separation. Additionally, standard medical textbooks from publishers such as Elsevier and Lippincott Williams and Wilkins were also referenced to encompass the latest advancements and established knowledge. This chapter shall explore the detailed anatomy of the neurovascular bundle, its clinical significance in ventral hernia repairs, and strategies to avoid damage and further complications.

2. Anatomy

2.1 Anterior abdominal wall

The anterior abdominal wall is a hexagonal area extending from the xiphoid process superiorly, coastal margins superolateral to the bilateral iliac crests and inguinal ligaments inferiorly, and the erector spinae and quadratus lumborum muscles inferiorly (**Figure 1**). The muscles within these boundaries function to alter intra-abdominal and intra-thoracic pressures, thereby assisting in respiration, coughing, defecation, and urination. Additionally, they exert a synergistic effect with the musculature of the back to facilitate flexion, extension, and rotation of the torso, produce tension of the thoracolumbar fascia, thus providing stabilization of the lumbosacral spine and pelvis, and hence play a critical role in maintaining posture [1].

The abdominal wall can be divided into two groups: the midline group of muscles and the anterolateral group of muscles. The midline group consists of the Rectus abdominis (RA) muscle and also the pyramidalis muscle in a small proportion of individuals. The anterolateral group consists of a trilaminar structure containing the external oblique (EO), internal oblique (IO), and transversus abdominis (TA) muscles (**Figure 2**).

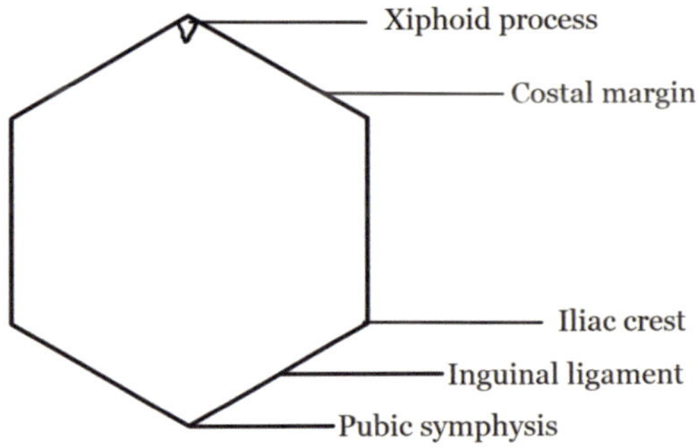

Figure 1.
Boundaries of anterior abdominal wall.

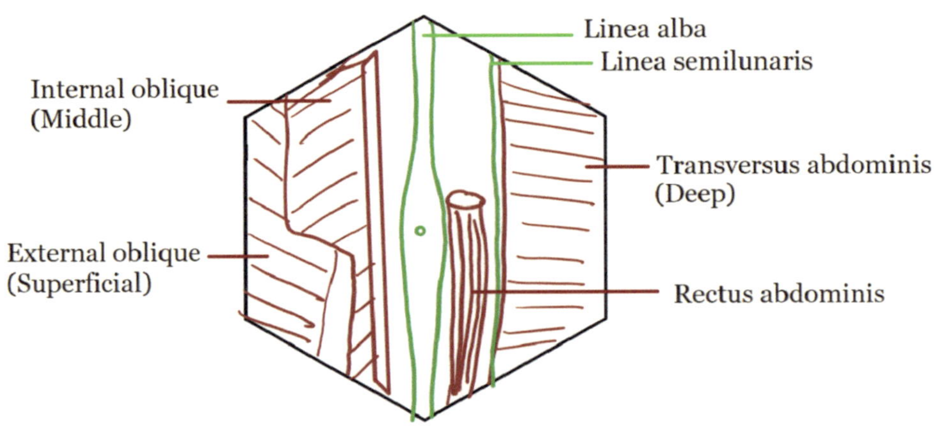

Figure 2.
Abdominal wall musculature.

	Above arcuate line	Below arcuate line
Anterior rectus sheath	1. External oblique aponeurosis 2. Anterior leaf of internal oblique aponeurosis	1. External oblique aponeurosis 2. Internal oblique aponeurosis 3. Tranversus abdominis aponeurosis
Posterior rectus sheath	1. Posterior leaf of internal oblique aponeurosis 2. Tranversus abdominis aponeurosis	Deficient

Table 1.
Derivations of anterior and posterior rectus sheath with respect to the arcuate line.

Linea alba is a completely fibrous structure running in the midline from the xiphoid process to the pubic symphysis (**Figure 2**). It is formed by the interlacing of the fibers of the aponeurosis of EO, IO, and TA muscles. It varies in it is width, being widest just above the umbilicus and narrowing at either end [2, 3]. It is the preferred site for surgical access to the abdomen due to its avascular nature, thus also making it a common site for incisional hernias. Also, the lack of musculature may lead to weakness and the formation of de novo ventral hernias. [4]

Linea semilunaris is noted by the insertion of EO, IO, and TA fascia at the lateral border of the RA muscle [4].

Rectus sheath is a flat aponeurotic compartment derived from EO, IO, and TA muscles, which enclose the RA muscle. It can be further divided into the anterior rectus sheath (ARS) and posterior rectus sheath (PRS), both inserted in the linea alba medially. The EO aponeurosis and anterior leaf of IO aponeurosis contribute to the ARS throughout it is length, whereas the posterior leaf of IO aponeurosis and the TA aponeurosis form the PRS. The arcuate line or semicircular line of Douglas is the anatomical landmark for the transition of the components of the PRS anterior to the RA muscle. Thus, below the arcuate line, the ARS is formed by the aponeurosis of all three anterolateral muscles, and the PRS is deficient with only the transversalis fascia between the RA and the peritoneum, thus representing an area with minimal strength (**Table 1**, **Figure 3A** and **B**) [5].

From a functional point of view, the abdominal wall can be divided into two components: anterior component (AC) and posterior component (PC) [6]. The AC includes the ARS and the rectus muscles, while the PC includes the PRS, transversalis fascia, and peritoneum.

2.2 Neurovascular bundle

The neurovascular bundle (NVB) comprises arteries, veins, and nerves lying in the retrorectus plane, that is, the plane between the rectus muscle and the posterior rectus sheath (**Figure 4**) [7, 8].

NVB can be divided into two components, namely, the neural structures, and the vasculature.

2.2.1 Neural structures

The nerves supplying the anterior abdominal wall and it is overlying skin are as follows:

a. Thoracoabdominal nerves:

These are derived from the anterior rami of the inferior six thoracic spinal nerves (T7–T11).

b. Subcostal nerve:

This nerve is the large anterior ramus of spinal nerve T12.

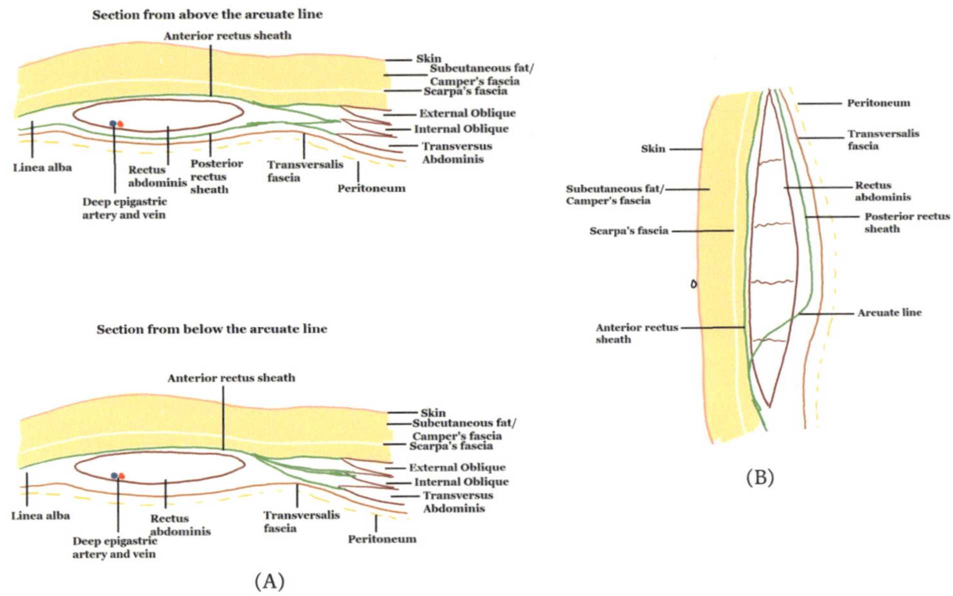

Figure 3.
A. Cross-sectional anatomy of rectus sheath. B. Sagittal section through rectus sheath.

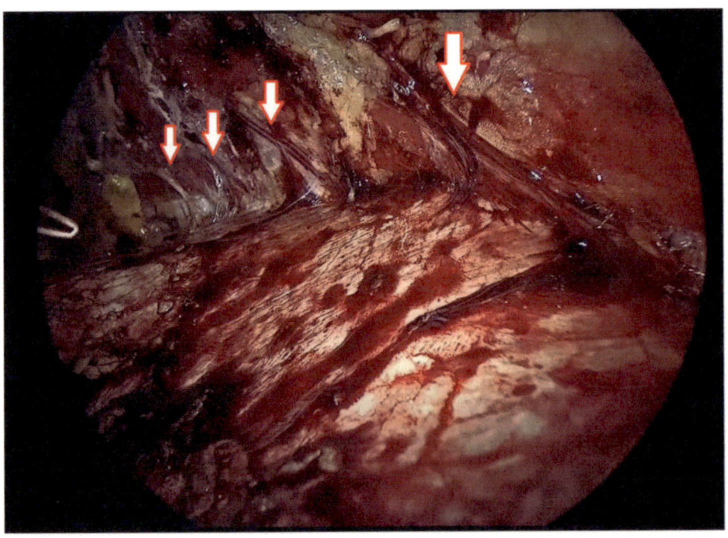

Figure 4.
Neurovascular bundles (Red arrows) as seen in a Laparoscopic extended view Totally extra-peritoneal (eTEP) ventral hernia repair.

c. Iliohypogastric and ilioinguinal nerves:

These are the terminal branches of the anterior ramus of spinal nerve L1 (**Table 2**). These nerves traverse the neurovascular plane between the internal oblique and transversus abdominis muscles in the lateral abdominal wall (**Figure 5**). They pierce the rectus sheath just medial to the linea semilunaris to enter the retrorectus space.

During their course through the anterolateral abdominal wall, the thoracoabdominal, subcostal, and iliohypogastric nerves communicate with each other.

2.2.2 Vasculature

The vessels supplying the anterior abdominal wall are as follows:

a. Superior epigastric artery

b. Inferior epigastric artery

c. Last six intercostal vessels

d. Four lumbar arteries

e. Deep circumflex iliac arteries

The superior epigastric artery, one of the terminal branches of the internal mammary artery, runs inferiorly in the rectus sheath to anatomose with inferior epigastric artery branches. It supplies the rectus abdominis muscle and the abdominal wall of the epigastric and upper umbilical regions.

The inferior epigastric artery arises from the external iliac artery just proximal to the inguinal ligament and runs superiorly in the transversalis fascia to enter the rectus sheath at the arcuate line. It supplies the rectus abdominis muscle and the deep abdominal wall of pubic and inferior umbilical regions (**Figure 6A** and **B**).

The deep circumflex iliac artery derived from the lateral part of the external iliac artery ascends to penetrate the abdominal wall musculature near the anterior superior iliac spine. It supplies the iliacus muscle, deep abdominal wall of the inguinal region, and iliac fossa.

The intercostal and lumbar arteries, the course between the transversus abdominis and internal oblique, along with nerves of the abdominal wall with their distal-most

Nerves	Origin	Distribution
Thoracoabdominal nerves	T7-T11	Anterolateral abdominal wall musculature and it is overlying skin
Subcostal nerve	T12	Anterolateral abdominal wall musculature and overlying skin between umbilicus and iliac crest
Iliohypogastric	L1	Skin overlying iliac crest, upper inguinal, and hypogastric regions; internal oblique and transversus abdominis muscles
Ilioinguinal	L1	Skin overlying inferior inguinal region, mons pubis, anterior scrotum or labium majus and adjacent medial thigh; inferior most internal oblique and transversus abdominis muscles

Table 2.
Nerves of the anterior abdominal wall.

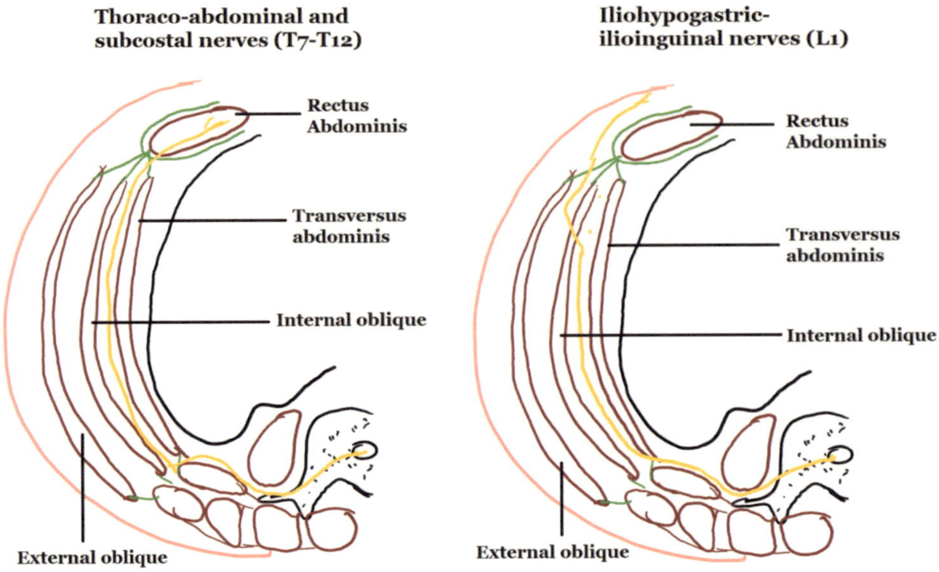

Figure 5.
Nerves of anterior abdominal wall.

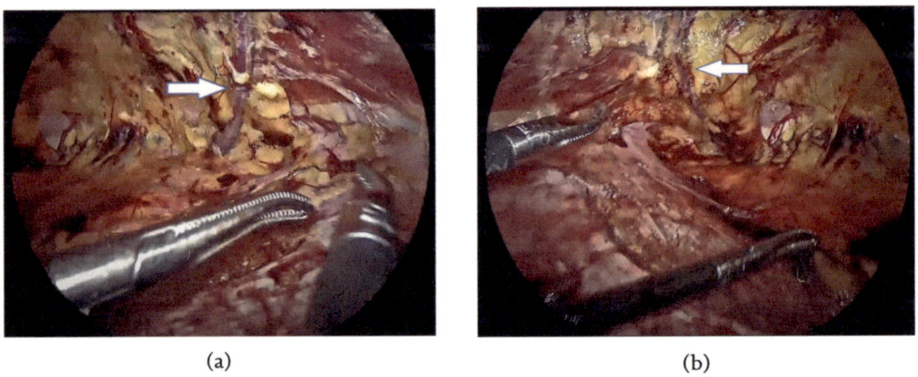

Figure 6.
A. Right inferior epigastric artery (Blue arrow). B. Left inferior epigastric artery (Blue arrow).

parts piercing the rectus sheath at different levels, medial to the linea semilunaris, communicate with the superior and inferior epigastric arteries.

Huger divided the vasculature into the three zones as follows (**Figure** 7).

1. Zone I/Superomedial: Superior epigastric arteries and deep inferior epigastric arteries supplying the upper midline RA with its overlying subcutaneous tissues and skin.

2. Zone II/Caudal: Superficial inferior epigastric and superficial external pudendal arteries supplying superficial fascia and skin in the lower abdomen along with deep inferior epigastric arteries and deep circumflex iliac arteries supplying the musculature in this region.

3. Zone II/Lateral: Lumbar and intercoastal arteries supplying the area lateral to linea semilunaris.

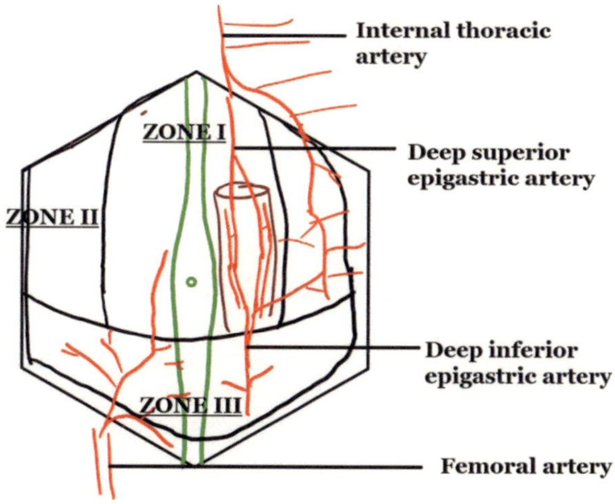

Figure 7.
Vascular supply of anterior abdominal wall showing Huger zones I-III.

3. Clinical significance

A thorough understanding of the anatomy and function of each component of the abdominal wall is essential before undertaking its repair or reconstruction in order to maintain and restore the functions of the abdominal wall following surgery. The restoration of linea alba helps maintain the function and integrity of the abdominal wall. Hence, the goal of abdominal wall reconstructions is restoring the linea alba by bringing the rectus muscles back to the midline. This has been shown to improve the isokinetic and isometric function of the abdominal wall, thereby improving quality of life postoperatively [9].

Preventing injuries to the NVB is of utmost importance while performing component separation hernia repairs via minimally invasive techniques (laparoscopic or robotic) as well as during open repairs.

Due to the overlapping innervation, damage to a few small branches may not impair the nervous supply considerably. However, damage to the larger nerves may lead to the weakening of the anterior abdominal wall, which would paradoxically lead to a lax abdominal wall with an increased risk of hernia formation.

Structure	Consequence of damage
Linea alba	Impaired function and integrity of abdominal wall
Nerves of anterior abdominal wall	Weakening and laxity of abdominal wall Loss of function of abdominal wall Recurrent hernias Abdominal bulges Asymmetry
Vasculature of anterior abdominal wall	Skin necrosis Hematoma formation

Table 3.
Impact of damage to various anatomical structures.

Abdominal wall vasculature comprises an extensive anastomotic blood supply. Damage to the superficial vasculature due to multiple surgical incisions may lead to skin necrosis postoperatively. Damage to deep vessels may lead to a hematoma formation, which may necessitate a surgical evacuation to avoid an increased risk of sepsis. The impact of damage to various anatomical structures has been summarized in **Table 3**.

4. Surgical techniques for NVB preservation

A thorough knowledge of the anatomy and it is correct identification is essential for a good surgical outcome. The distorted anatomy of recurrent hernia repairs might make the identification of the NVB more challenging owing to the adhesions and fibrosis that ensue due to the previous surgery. Furthermore, anatomical variations may also pose a challenge to the accurate identification of the NVB.

4.1 Surgical techniques for ventral hernia repair

The traditional onlay mesh repair popularized by Chevrel in 1979 involves placement of the mesh on the sutured anterior rectus fascia below the subcutaneous tissue [10]. The sublay mesh technique involves placing the mesh in the retrorectus plane. This technique was introduced in 1965 by Rene Stoppa, who placed the mesh in the pre-peritoneal or the retrofascial space. Further, in 1966, Jean Rives advocated placing the mesh in the retromuscular plane, that is, below the rectus muscle and above the PRS, thus popularizing the use of this retromuscular technique for ventral hernia repairs [11, 12]. This technique revolutionized hernia repairs by giving good surgical outcomes and low recurrence rates [13].

Separation of components was initially described by Ramirez in 1990 as a technique to increase the laxity of the abdominal wall to facilitate a tension-free repair [14]. While it was originally described without the use of a prosthetic mesh, it has since then evolved since then to include the use of an underlay mesh or retrorectus technique with mesh placement. Carbonell introduced the concept of posterior component separation in 2008, in which he divided the internal oblique fascia and dissected between the IO and TA to create space for mesh placement [15]. A major pitfall of this technique was the division of the neurovascular bundle, leading to lax abdominal wall, abdominal wall bulges, recurrent hernia, and asymmetry [16, 17].

A novel approach to posterior component separation was then introduced by Yuri Novitsky and Michael Rosen in 2012 [18, 19]. Their approach, called the transversus abdominis release (TAR), involved the extension of the retrorectus plane of Rives-Stoppa laterally by dividing attachments of the TA muscle. This technique proved to be a solution to the wound morbidity and mesh limitations of AC separation techniques while giving low perioperative morbidity and low recurrence rates.

The first laparoscopic ventral hernia repair was described by Le Blanc and Booth in 1993, which involved placing a mesh intra-peritoneally and fixing it to the anterior abdominal wall [20]. The new era of laparoscopic surgery ushered in laparoscopic techniques of component separation. In 2000, Dr. Lowe and colleagues described the first laparoscopic anterior component separation, whereas Igor Belyanksy described laparoscopic TAR in 2016 [21, 22].

4.2 Surgical strategies for preservation of NVB

The surgical linchpin for the conservation of NVB is used to avoid the plane between the internal oblique and transversus abdominis muscles, which contains the neurovascular bundle. Component separation techniques, which have ushered in a new era for ventral hernia repairs, either access the plane between external and internal oblique muscles (anterior component separation) or the plane between transversus abdominis and transversalis fascia (posterior component separation), thus avoiding the neurovascular plane.

Another common area of NVB injury is at the segmental NVB during retrorectus and posterior component separation repairs, where the NVB pierces the rectus sheath just medial to the linea semilunaris. It is essential to carefully identify the NVB at this stage. It may be advisable to supplement this step with the use of adjuncts such as indocyanine green (ICG) dye to visualize the exact location of the NVB and hence prevent an accidental injury (**Figures 8** and **9**; Video 1, https://drive.google.com/file/d/1kQ_UfjKUqSDFX2676ghaiu8Bh9Np5hc-/view?usp=drive_web) [23]. This maybe vital in recurrent cases and anatomical variations, where identification of the NVB is especially challenging.

In the posterior component separation technique, that is, Transversus abdominis release (TAR), we recommend incising the rectus sheath about 1 cm medial to the

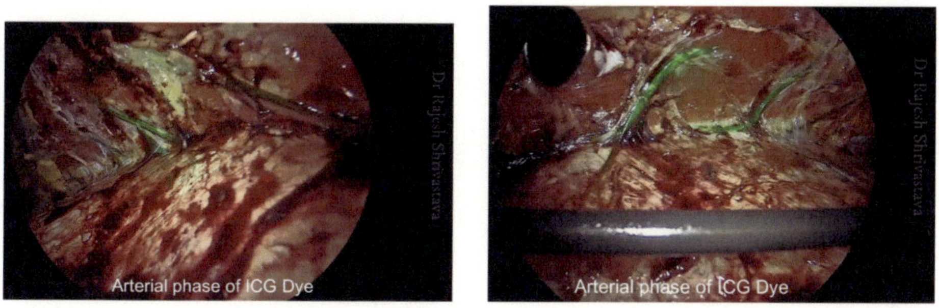

(a) (b)

Figure 8.
A. Neurovascular bundles in the arterial phase of indocyanine green dye on the right side. B. Neurovascular bundles in the arterial phase of indocyanine green dye on the left side.

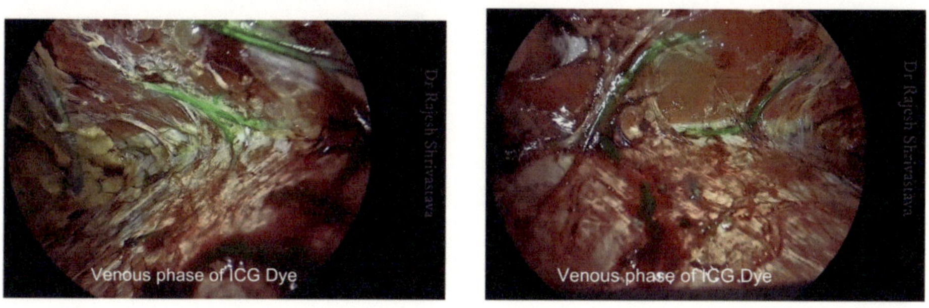

(a) (b)

Figure 9.
A. Neurovascular bundles in the venous phase of indocyanine green dye on the right side. B. Neurovascular bundles in the venous phase of indocyanine green dye on the left side.

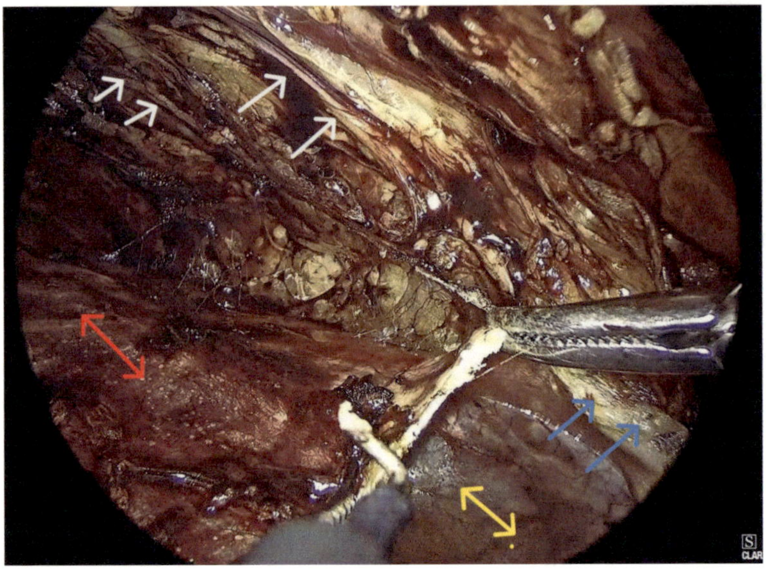

Figure 10.
Transversus Abdominis Release in process. White arrows: Neurovascular bundle. Blue arrows: Divided transversus abdominis muscle. Yellow arrow: Peritoneum. Red arrow: Posterior rectus sheath.

linea semilunaris to adequately preserve the NVB and reduce any further difficulties while placing the mesh (**Figure 10**).

Adequate hemostasis in case of inadvertent vascular injury with a bipolar energy device is a must to avoid postoperative hematoma formation.

5. Conclusion

The neurovascular bundle plays a pivotal role in ventral hernia repairs. An in-depth understanding of its anatomy and proper identification are essential to avoid iatrogenic damage to the NVB. Careful, meticulous dissection and preservation of the NVB may help reduce debilitating postoperative complications and in turn lead to improved patient outcomes and quality of life.

DOI: http://dx.doi.org/10.5772/intechopen.1006503

Author details

Rajesh Shrivastava[1,2]* and Nazrah Shaikh[3]

1 Vedanta Institute of Medical Sciences, Maharashtra, India

2 Shreeji Hospital, India

3 Sir H. N. Reliance Foundation Hospital, Mumbai, India

*Address all correspondence to: dr.rajeshshree70@gmail.com

References

[1] Willard FH, Vleeming A, Schuenke MD, Danneels L, Schleip R. The thoracolumbar fascia: Anatomy, function and clinical considerations. Journal of Anatomy. 2012;**221**(6):507-536

[2] Rath AM, Attali P, Dumas JL, Goldlust D, Zhang J, Chevrel JP. The abdominal linea alba: An anatomo-radiologic and biomechanical study. Surgical and Radiologic Anatomy. 1996;**18**(4):281-288

[3] Beer GM, Schuster A, Seifert B, Manestar M, Mihic Probst D, Weber SA. The normal width of the linea alba in nulliparous women. Clinical Anatomy. 2009;**22**(6):706-711

[4] Johnson TG, Von SJ, Hope WW. Clinical anatomy of the abdominal wall: Hernia surgery. OA Anatomy. 2014;**2**(1):3

[5] Montgomery A, Petersson U, Austrums E. The arcuate line hernia: Operative treatment and a review of the literature. Hernia. 2013;**17**:391-396

[6] Cavalli M, Bruni PG, Lombardo F, Morlacchi A, Andretto Amodeo C, Campanelli G. Original concepts in anatomy, abdominal-wall surgery, and component separation technique and strategy. Hernia. 2020;**24**(2):411-419. DOI: 10.1007/s10029-019-02030-7. Epub 2019 Sep 6

[7] Townsend JCM, Beauchamp RD, Evers BM, Mattox KL. Sabiston Textbook of Surgery. 21st ed. Philadelphia, PA: Elsevier - Health Sciences Division; 2021

[8] Moore KL, Dalley AF, Agur A. Clinically Oriented Anatomy. 9th ed. Philadelphia, PA: Lippincott Williams and Wilkins; 2023

[9] Criss CN, Petro CC, Krpata DM, Seafler CM, Lai N, Fiutem J, et al. Functional abdominal wall reconstruction improves core physiology and quality-of-life. Surgery. 2014;**156**(1):176-182

[10] Chevrel JP. Traitement des grandes éventrations médianes par plastie en paletot et prothèse [the treatment of large midline incisional hernias by "overcoat" plasty and prothesis (author's transl)]. La Nouvelle Presse Médicale. 1979;**8**(9):695-696. French

[11] Rives J, Lardennois B, Pire JC, Hibon J, Large incisional hernias. The importance of flail abdomen and of subsequent respiratory disorders. Chirurgie. 1973;**99**(8):547-563

[12] Stoppa RE. The treatment of complicated groin and incisional hernias. World Journal of Surgery. 1989;**13**(5):545-554

[13] Iqbal CW, Pham TH, Joseph A, Mai J, Thompson GB, Sarr MG. Long-term outcome of 254 complex incisional hernia repairs using the modified Rives-Stoppa technique. World Journal of Surgery. 2007;**31**(12):2398-2404

[14] Ramirez OM, Ruas E, Dellon AL. "Components separation" method for closure of abdominal wall defects: An anatomic and clinical study. Plastic and Reconstructive Surgery. 1990;**86**:519

[15] Carbonell AM, Cobb WS, Chen SM. Posterior components separation during retromuscular hernia repair. Hernia. 2008;**12**(4):359-362

[16] Kumar S, Edmunds RW, Dowdy C, Chang YW, King R, et al. Anterior versus posterior component separation: Which

is better? Plastic and Reconstructive Surgery. 2018;**142**:47S-53S

[17] Siegal SR, Pauli EM. Posterior component separation/transversus abdominis release. Plastic and Aesthetic Research. 2019;**6**:25

[18] Novitsky YW, Fayezizadeh M, Majumder A, Neupane R, Elliott HL, Orenstein SB. Outcomes of posterior component separation with transversus abdominis muscle release and synthetic mesh sublay reinforcement. Annals of Surgery. 2016;**264**(2):226-232

[19] Novitsky YW. Posterior component separation via transversus abdominis muscle release: The TAR procedure. In: Hernia Surgery. Switzerland: Springer International; 2016. pp. 117-135

[20] LeBlanc KA, Booth WV. Laparoscopic repair of incisional abdominal hernias using expanded polytetrafluoroethylene: Preliminary findings. Surgical Laparoscopy & Endoscopy. Feb 1993;**3**(1):39-41

[21] Lowe JB, Garza JR, Bowman JL, Rohrich RJ, Strodel WE. Endoscopically assisted "components separation" for closure of abdominal wall defects. Plastic and Reconstructive Surgery. 2000;**105**(2):720-730

[22] Belyansky I, Zahiri HR, Park A. Laparoscopic Transversus abdominis release, a novel minimally invasive approach to complex Abdominal Wall reconstruction. Surgical Innovation. 2016;**23**(2):134-141

[23] Aarsh G, Jignesh G, Shrivastava R. The role of indocyanine green fluorescence angiography in ventral hernia repair. Hernia. 2024. DOI: 10.1007/s10029-024-03014-y

Chapter 3

Enhanced-View Totally Extraperitoneal Approach to Retrorectus Ventral Hernia Repair

August Schaeffer and Richard Lu

Abstract

The field of abdominal wall reconstruction is a rapidly growing field. New methods of hernia repair are being developed, and multiple platforms, including robotics, are now being used for the treatment of complex hernias. One such novel surgical technique is the enhanced-view totally extraperitoneal (eTEP) approach to ventral hernia repair. Advantages of this technique include dynamic access to the retrorectus space in an extraperitoneal fashion that allows for large mesh overlap in a well vascularized tissue plane. The retrorectus repair has a low rate of recurrence and with the advantages of a minimally invasive approach including decreased postoperative pain and duration of hospitalisation. This chapter provides an outline on patient selection, operative techniques, and postoperative care.

Keywords: robotic surgery, extraperitoneal retrorectus repair, enhanced-view totally extraperitoneal approach, eTEP, ventral hernia herniorrhaphy, minimally invasive abdominal wall reconstruction

1. Introduction

The field of abdominal wall reconstruction has rapidly evolved in recent years with a trend towards increased use of minimally invasive techniques and extraperitoneal mesh placement [1, 2]. The retrorectus repairs, both open and laparoscopic, have an established low rate of recurrence [3]. Studies have shown decreased rates of postoperative pain and hospital stay compared to laparoscopic intraperitoneal onlay mesh (IPOM) repairs, despite the more extensive dissection [4, 5]. Described by Belyansky and colleagues, the enhanced-view totally extraperitoneal (eTEP) ventral hernia repair represents a novel minimally invasive approach to retromuscular ventral hernia repair [6]. Utilization of retromuscular hernia repair has gained increasing popularity given the ability to provide wide mesh overlap in a vascular rich space without direct contact with underlying intraabdominal viscera. The focus of this chapter is to provide a comprehensive understanding of an eTEP retrorectus ventral hernia repair.

2. Preoperative planning

As with any operation, appropriate patient evaluation and selection is key to success. A thorough history and physical examination should be performed. It is critical to obtain a detailed surgical history, as many hernias originate from incisions of prior operations. Prior operative reports can provide invaluable information, particularly those of prior hernia repairs when managing a recurrent hernia. Medical comorbidities such as diabetes, smoking, and diabetes should be identified. Any reversible comorbidity should be optimized as best as possible prior to offering surgical intervention. The physical exam should include assessment and documentation of the size and location of the hernia. Past surgical incisions should be noted, along with wounds and any other soft tissue abnormalities.

Imaging studies such as computed tomography (CT) of the abdominal wall should be considered for operative planning. Imaging provides information of the hernia contents, defect size, and anatomical details of the abdominal wall such as rectus width. There are several factors that are important in selecting an appropriate candidate for eTEP. The hallmark maneuver of eTEP is the crossover maneuver, which relies on the adipose rich preperitoneal space in the midline. Previous manipulation of this space from prior surgery, particularly from large midline incisions, can disrupt this space and preclude eTEP. Little to no midline preperitoneal fat on CT imaging, particularly in a patient with history of a midline incision, may predict a difficult crossover.

3. Operative approach

3.1 Patient positioning and retrorectus access

The patient is positioned supine with the arms tucked. The hips of the patient should be aligned with the break of the bed to allow flexion of the operating table, which expands the distance between the anterior superior iliac spine and the costal margin. Access to the retrorectus space is performed with either optical trocar or direct cutdown technique. The decision on which retrorectus space is used for initial access is determined by history of any prior operations that may disrupt native anatomy. For example, if a patient had history of colostomy placement with subsequent reversal over the left abdomen, the right retrorectus space should be accessed. Retrorectus access is typically achieved just below the costal margin as there is less abdominal wall compliance in this region, which facilitates more accurate entry. While placing the trocar, each layer of the abdominal wall should be visualized. Once the anterior rectus sheath is encountered, the surgeon should anticipate the rectus abdominus muscle directly below (**Figure 1**).

The muscle fibers of the rectus abdominis are swept away with the tip of the trocar and endoscope, exposing the posterior rectus sheath. Once the posterior rectus sheath is encountered, the angle of the trocar and endoscope should be made more shallow, aligning the direction of dissection parallel to the retrorectus plane. This facilitates efficient dissection of the retrorectus space and prevents accidental injury to the posterior rectus sheath, which leads to collapse of the space due to insufflation leaking into the intraperitoneal space. The retrorectus space should then be developed by bluntly dissecting through the areolar tissue between the posterior rectus sheath and the rectus muscle. Care should be taken to avoid avulsing branches of the epigastric

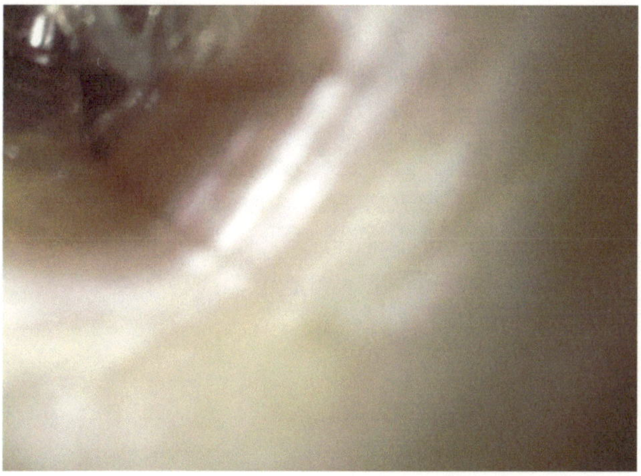

Figure 1.
Entry into the rectus sheath with visualization of the rectus muscle fibers. From superficial to deep, the subcutaneous adipose tissue can be visualized followed by the anterior rectus sheath and underlying rectus abdominis muscle.

Hernia defect location	Recommended port position	Relative contraindications to port placement
Upper midline	Lower or lateral abdomen	Previous pelvic surgery or morbid obesity with large pannus
Lower midline	Upper or lateral abdomen	Previous upper midline or subcostal incisions
Paraumbilical	Lateral abdomen	Retrorectus space less than 7 cm

Table 1.
Port placement and relative contraindications.

arteries; instead, they should be carefully dissected off the posterior sheath. Blunt endoscopic dissection continues until there is adequate room to place additional trocars. An advantage of the eTEP technique is dynamic port placement. Depending on the location of the hernia, ports may be placed in the upper, lower, or lateral abdomen. Although this chapter's figures are sourced from a robotic case, a similar concept of port placement selection can be applied to standard laparoscopy. **Table 1** lists port placement options and the relative contraindications for each setup.

The retrorectus space is developed medially to the insertion of the posterior rectus sheath to linea alba, and laterally to the linea semilunaris where the neurovascular bundles are visualized (**Figure 2**).

3.2 The crossover maneuver

The crossover maneuver is the defining step of the eTEP technique during which the bilateral retrorectus spaces are joined with the medial preperitoneal space in an extraperitoneal fashion. The preperitoneal adipose tissue from the falciform and umbilical ligaments are critical anatomic structures for this maneuver. Disruption of these elements from prior surgeries may complicate the crossover. Thus, the decision to crossover in either the upper or lower abdomen is based on prior disruption to this space. For example, a history of pelvic or lower abdominal surgeries may warrant an

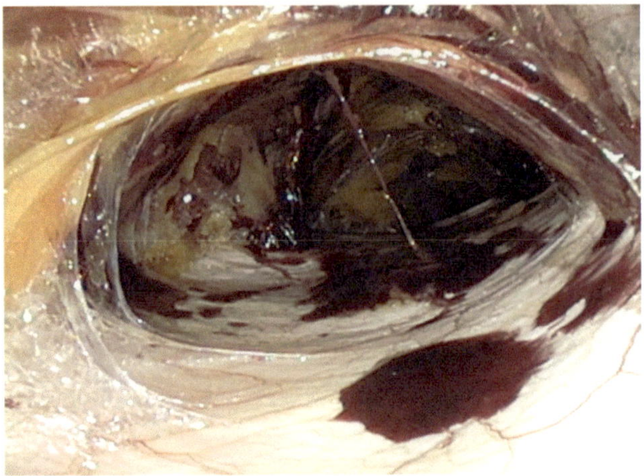

Figure 2.
The retrorectus space can be mostly developed with blunt dissection. The posterior rectus sheath is seen below and the rectus abdominis muscle above. Structures such as the neurovascular bundles and inferior epigastric vessels course along the muscle and is usually covered with adipose tissue.

upper crossover utilizing the falciform ligament, whereas an epigastric hernia may be better addressed with a lower crossover with the umbilical ligaments.

The interface of the medial aspect of the posterior rectus sheath where it joins with the anterior rectus sheath to form linea alba should be identified. An incision is made on the medial aspect of the posterior rectus sheath approximately 0.5 cm away from the linea alba to avoid accidental injury to this critical structure. Once the medial aspect of the posterior rectus sheath is incised, the underlying preperitoneal fat from either the falciform or umbilical ligaments are encountered (**Figure 3**).

The preperitoneal fat is dissected off the linea alba until the contralateral posterior rectus sheath is encountered. Identification of the contralateral posterior rectus sheath can be difficult. The shadow of the contralateral rectus muscle can typically be seen, and a short burst of monopolar energy inducing muscle twitch can help identify

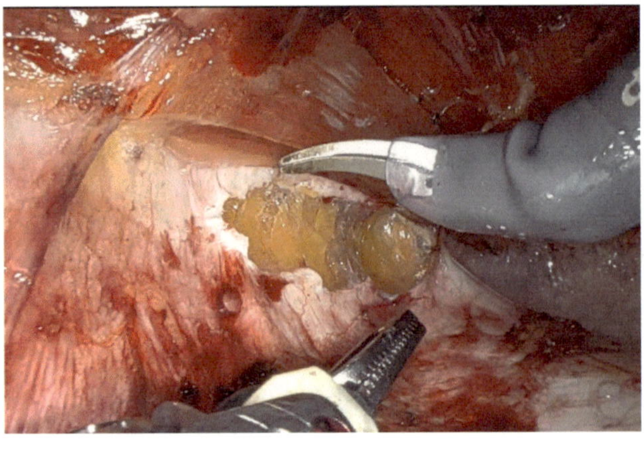

Figure 3.
The crossover maneuver is initiated by incising the medial aspect of the posterior rectus sheath, exposing the underlying midline preperitoneal fat.

the correct location. In addition, the lack of decussating fibers on the contralateral posterior rectus sheath in contrast to the linea alba can also help identify anatomy (**Figure 4**).

The contralateral posterior rectus sheath is then incised and the underlying contralateral rectus abdominis muscle is encountered, marking the completion of the crossover maneuver. The midline dissection continues such that the entire linea alba, including any hernia defects, are exposed (**Figure 5**). It is important to remember that eTEP is an approach to retromuscular hernia repair. Depending on the complexity of the hernia, the intraperitoneal space may need to be entered to safely reduce the hernia contents. The remainder of the retrorectus space is developed to the contralateral linea semilunaris as marked by the neurovascular bundles (**Figure 6**). From this space, a transversus abdominis release (TAR) can be performed if necessary. The technical details of TAR are beyond the scope of this chapter.

3.3 Closure of hernia defects and mesh placement

The linea alba is then plicated to address any diastasis recti and the hernia defects are incorporated into the suture line, typically with 0 absorbable barbed suture (**Figure 7**). Although approximation of the posterior sheaths is not necessary, the authors will proceed with closure of the posterior rectus sheath if there is no excessive tension. If tension on the posterior layer exists, bridging peritoneum is adequate. In rare cases, large posterior layer defects may require bridging with an absorbable mesh. A transversus abdominis release can be considered for more laxity on the posterior layer, but should only be utilized as a last resort. Mesh is trimmed to size and placed within the retromuscular space (**Figure 8**). The authors use a medium weight macroporous polypropylene mesh trimmed to fit the retrorectus space. Fixation is typically not necessary, however, if issues exist in keeping the mesh flat, interrupted absorbable sutures to secure the mesh can be considered. Although some studies have shown that retromuscular drains have been shown to decrease the rate of retromuscular seroma, drainage should be considered on a case-to-case basis. The abdomen

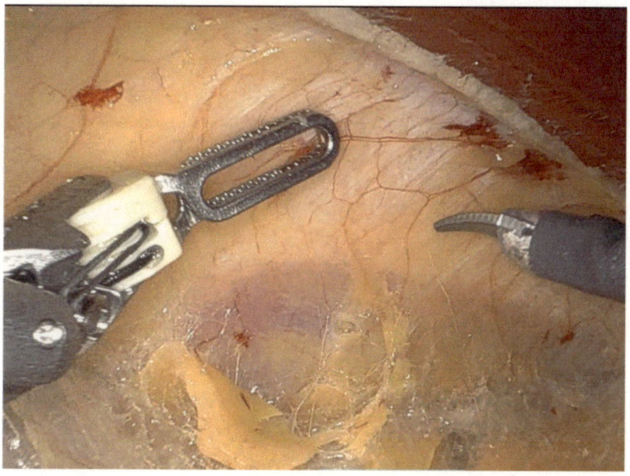

Figure 4.
Exposure of the linea alba is obtained by clearing off the preperitoneal fat and reducing all midline hernia defects. The shadow of the contralateral rectus abdominis muscle can be seen. When entering the contralateral retrorectus space, it is important to prevent accidental injury to the linea alba.

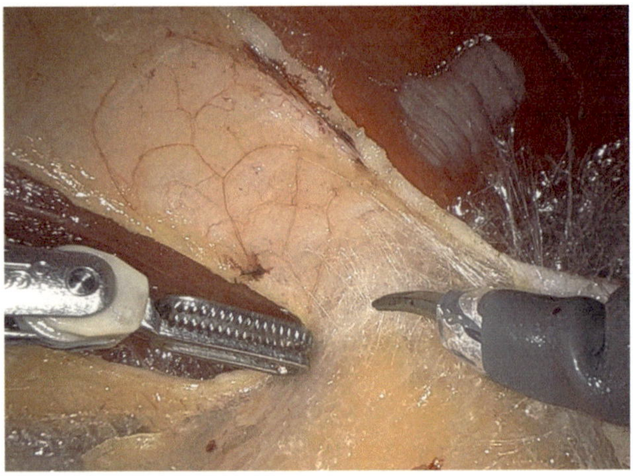

Figure 5.
The crossover is completed by incising the contralateral posterior rectus sheath, exposing the contralateral rectus abdominis muscle. In this photo, the linea alba is seen devoid of preperitoneal fat with both rectus muscles seen laterally.

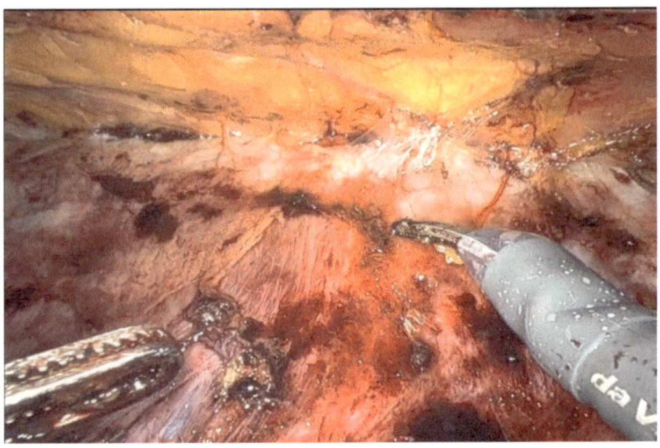

Figure 6.
The retrorectus space is developed to its most lateral extent, the linea semilunaris. Neurovascular bundles are typically seen exiting medial to the linea semilunaris to provide innervation to the rectus abdominis muscles.

is then desufflated under direct visualization to ensure hemostasis and satisfactory placement of the mesh.

4. Postoperative care

Most patients who undergo eTEP Rives-Stoppa repair can be discharged the same day. If retromuscular drains were placed, they are typically removed in 1 to 2 weeks once output approaches 30 cc/day. Activity should be progressed slowly as tolerated by the patient.

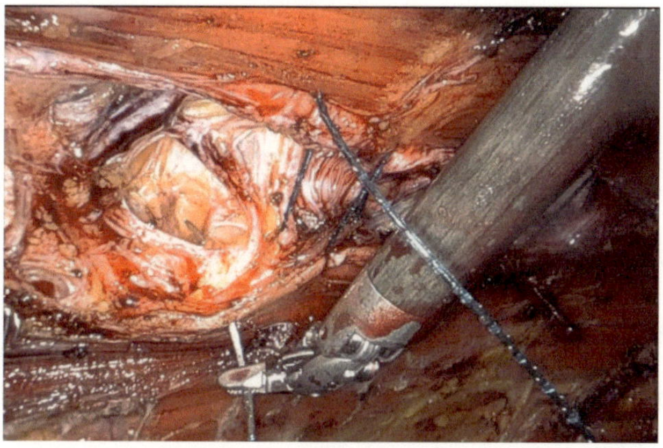

Figure 7.
The hernia defects are closed with barbed suture.

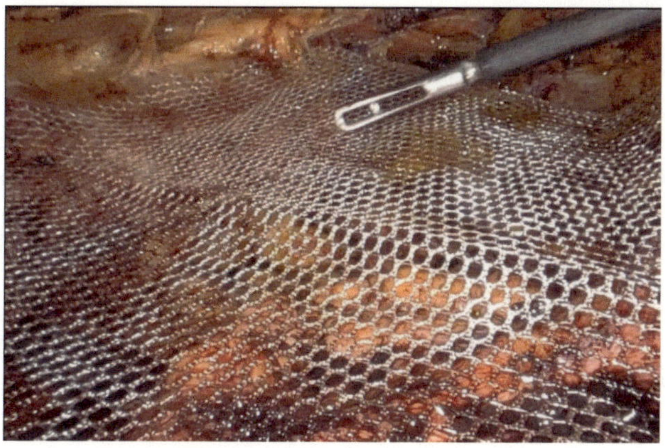

Figure 8.
A polypropylene mesh is placed within the rectus abdominis space.

5. Postoperative complications

5.1 Fluid collections

The most common complications of eTEP are the development of postoperative fluid collections such as hematomas and seromas [7]. Hematomas typically occur from inadequate hemostasis, usually from a branch from the epigastric vessels or neurovascular bundles. Abdominal wall ecchymosis with increased abdominal bulging may be signs of a postoperative retromuscular hematoma. A discrete mass may not be present due to anterior rectus sheath containing the hematoma. A strong suspicion of a retromuscular hematoma should prompt blood work and CT imaging. Hematomas that cause hemodynamic changes or present with active contrast extravasation on CT imaging must be surgical explored urgently for hematoma evacuation. However, most hematomas are small and can be observed. Large symptomatic hematomas should be considered for hematoma evacuation to improve the patient's clinical presentation and prevent the hematoma from interfering with mesh integration. Postoperative seromas following eTEP may be either subcutaneous or retromuscular. Small seromas can be observed, however, large and symptomatic hernias should be aspirated. Seromas refractory to aspiration and drain placement may need repeat therapy, and in rare cases, surgical excision.

5.2 Posterior layer dehiscence

One of the most devastating complications of eTEP is breakdown of the posterior layers creating an intraparietal hernia. These can present as postoperative bowel obstruction with CT imaging demonstrating herniation of intraperitoneal contents through the layers of the abdominal wall. Posterior layer dehiscence in the early postoperative period should undergo diagnostic laparoscopy with reduction of the contents and repair of the posterior layer defect, typically with an IPOM approach.

5.3 Anterior layer dehiscence

Dehiscence of the anterior fascial closure may present as a recurrent midline abdominal bulge. The timing and extent of dehiscence is critical in tailoring the management of this complication. If dehiscence is noticed in the operating room, typically during emergence from anesthesia, the surgeon should proceed with surgical exploration to repair the suture line. Early large postoperative anterior fascial dehiscence should also be brought back to the operating room for exploration and repair. Small postoperative anterior sheath dehiscence may be observed.

The most dreaded complication is a complete blowout of the repair, with failure of both the anterior and posterior layers. These patients typically present with an acute abdomen and warrant urgent surgical exploration. Resection of non-viable viscera should be performed if present and formal abdominal wall reconstruction deferred to a later time.

6. Conclusion

The eTEP approach to retromuscular ventral hernia repair is another valuable tool in a hernia surgeon's armamentarium. This extraperitoneal retromuscular approach offers dynamic port placement within a versatile anatomic plane for management of ventral hernias. A strong understanding of abdominal wall anatomy and careful preoperative planning are imperative for the success of this novel and versatile technique.

Author details

August Schaeffer and Richard Lu*
The University of Texas Medical Branch in Galveston, Galveston, TX, USA

*Address all correspondence to: rllu@utmb.edu

References

[1] Madion M, Goldblatt MI, Gould JC, Higgins RM. Ten-year trends in minimally invasive hernia repair: A NSQIP database review. Surgical Endoscopy. 2021;**35**(12):7200-7208. DOI: 10.1007/s00464-020-08217-9

[2] Howard R, Thumma J, Ehlers A, Englesbe M, Dimick J, Telem D. Trends in surgical technique and outcomes of ventral hernia repair in the United States. Annals of Surgery. 2023;**278**(2):274-279. DOI: 10.1097/SLA.0000000000005654

[3] Den Hartog FPJ, Sneiders D, Darwish EF, et al. Favorable outcomes after retro-rectus (rives-stoppa) mesh repair as treatment for noncomplex ventral abdominal wall hernia, a systematic review and meta-analysis. Annals of Surgery. 2022;**276**(1):55-65. DOI: 10.1097/SLA.0000000000005422

[4] Jensen KK, Helgstrand F, Henriksen NA. Short-term outcomes after laparoscopic IPOM versus robot-assisted retromuscular repair of small to medium ventral hernias: A nationwide database study. Annals of Surgery. 2024;**279**(1):154-159. DOI: 10.1097/SLA.0000000000005915

[5] Christoffersen MW, Jørgensen LN, Jensen KK. Less postoperative pain and shorter length of stay after robot-assisted retrorectus hernia repair (rRetrorectus) compared with laparoscopic intraperitoneal onlay mesh repair (IPOM) for small or medium-sized ventral hernias. Surgical Endoscopy. 2023;**37**(2):1053-1059. DOI: 10.1007/s00464-022-09608-w

[6] Belyansky I, Daes J, Radu VG, et al. A novel approach using the enhanced-view totally extraperitoneal (eTEP) technique for laparoscopic retromuscular hernia repair. Surgical Endoscopy. 2018;**32**(3):1525-1532. DOI: 10.1007/s00464-017-5840-2

[7] Mazzola Poli de Figueiredo S, Belyansky I, Lu R. Pitfalls and complications of enhanced-view totally extraperitoneal approach to abdominal wall reconstruction. Surgical Endoscopy. 2023;**37**(5):3354-3363. DOI: 10.1007/s00464-022-09843-1

Chapter 4

Parastomal Hernia: From Definitions and Management to Prevention

Adam Daniel Gerrard and Raimundas Lunevicius

Abstract

Parastomal hernias are a common complication of ostomy formation, with end colostomies twice as likely to develop parastomal hernias. Older age, high body mass index, synchronous chronic diseases, collagen deficit disorders, and medication use increase the risk of parastomal hernia development. Whilst many hernias can be appreciated clinically, computed tomography has an important preoperative role in hernia assessment and treatment planning. Parastomal hernia repair method depends on patient factors, the surgeon's skill set, the surgical setting where the hernia repair takes place, and the presence or absence of concomitant midline incisional hernia. Where there is no midline incisional hernia, the Sugarbaker technique, minimally invasive or open, is advised. A posterior component separation technique is recommended to repair the parastomal defect when a parastomal hernia is large and (or) there is a midline incisional hernia. There are reported benefits of the laparoscopic approach over open parastomal hernia repair, such as reduced risk of postoperative complications and recurrence. The risk of parastomal hernia occurrence in elective end colostomies may be reduced using prophylactic mesh.

Keywords: parastomal hernia, colostomy, ileostomy, urostomy, hernia repair, hernia prevention, stoma, risk factors, abdominal wall reconstruction, hernia mesh

1. Introduction

By virtue of fashioning an ostomy through the abdominal wall, an inherent weakness is created. Therefore, both large and small bowel ostomies are associated with high parastomal hernia rates. The consequences of parastomal hernia for the patient can vary from cosmetic dissatisfaction and difficulty adhering the ostomy bag to the surrounding skin to pain, intestinal obstruction, and acute bowel strangulation. A parastomal hernia may be encountered by the specialised abdominal wall surgeon, but also the emergency general surgeon on call and the colorectal or urological surgeon responsible for creating the stoma.

This chapter will review the definitions, incidence, risk factors, diagnosis, classification, and management of parastomal hernias. It will also review the methods of preventing their formation, ranging from modifiable patient factors to ostomy site selection, surgical technique, and prophylactic adjuncts.

2. Definitions

A parastomal hernia is an incisional hernia in which abdominal contents protrude through the surgical site where an ostomy was created. A colonic or small bowel ostomy may be formed for various benign or malignant pathologies. First described in the sixteenth century [1], the creation of such ostomies is one of the most commonly performed surgeries in both elective and emergency settings for benign and malignant diseases. Intestinal stomas can be formed from the large (colostomy) or small bowel, which may divert bowel content (jejunostomy or ileostomy) or urine (urostomy). Depending upon their indication and related anatomy, stomas may be temporary or permanent.

Stomas are created by exteriorising the bowel through the abdominal wall. Often brought out through the rectus abdominis muscle, the formation of stoma results in loss of subcutaneous tissue, incision to the anterior rectus sheath, splitting of the rectus abdominis muscle, and finally, division of the posterior rectus sheath and parietal peritoneum. Whilst necessary for delivering the bowel to the surface, this dissection anatomically predisposes the abdominal wall to parastomal hernia formation.

3. Incidence

In the United Kingdom, it is estimated that 1 in 335 people have a stoma [2]. In the United States of America, 130,000 new stomas are created each year [3]. A parastomal hernia as an early postoperative complication is rare. The incidence of parastomal hernia increases over time, varying by stoma type and between reported studies, but can be estimated between 5% and 50% with colostomies twice more likely to have a parastomal hernia than an ileostomy [4–7].

4. Risk factors

Independent risk factors relating to patient characteristics and operative technique have been identified for parastomal hernia development. Older age at formation of stoma (>60 years) has been demonstrated to be associated with subsequent parastomal hernia [8, 9]. There have been conflicting reports on the effect of sex on the risk of parastomal hernia. A large Danish registry study concluded that the male sex carries an increased risk for parastomal hernia occurrence [9], whilst other studies and meta-analyses have deemed the female sex to be the more significant hazard in this respect [10–12]. Risk factors related to surgery include the formation of an end colostomy, laparoscopic approach, defect aperture over 3 cm in size, not delivering the stoma through the middle of the rectus abdominis muscle, and postoperative infection [13].

Further disease-related risk factors for parastomal hernia formation are diabetes mellitus, diverticulitis, cancer, liver cirrhosis, chronic obstructive pulmonary disease, benign prostatic hyperplasia, and collagen synthesis disorders [14, 15]. These conditions either affect wound healing and tissue strength or raise intra-abdominal pressures. There are potentially modifiable risk factors that increase the risk of parastomal hernia development. Patients with a high body mass index (BMI) and (or) large waist circumference are at increased risk of parastomal hernia due to the raised intra-abdominal pressure; this weakens the abdominal wall musculature [10, 16–18]. Patients who smoke, strain with chronic constipation, and (or) are taking steroid medication also have an increased risk of parastomal hernia occurrence.

5. Diagnosis

In the outpatient setting, patients with a parastomal hernia may be asymptomatic or present with symptoms of bulging around the stoma, which is exaggerated when coughing or moving. The subsequent bulging of the abdominal wall may have cosmetic consequences for the patient, and (or) they may struggle to get a good seal with their ostomy bag. Patients may experience abdominal discomfort around the parastomal hernia, particularly if it is large. Chronic skin changes may occur due to stretching or pressure effects.

In the acute surgery setting, patients may present with a hard and tender hernia, with the overlying skin becoming red or warmer. If the hernia is causing stoma obstruction, output from the ostomy may cease, and the patient will experience abdominal distention, pain, and vomiting. Strangulation of an incarcerated bowel loop within the hernia sac is a life-threatening complication of a parastomal hernia, which requires immediate surgical intervention.

Clinical assessment involves a comprehensive history that explores the indication for stoma formation and risk factors for parastomal hernia formation. Current hernia symptoms must be assessed, and patient concerns and expectations should be explored. In view of potential parastomal hernia repair, an assessment of general fitness for a surgical procedure should be undertaken.

The examination should focus on the whole abdomen. When planning parastomal hernia management, it is essential to assess any other hernia, particularly incisional from concurrent midline laparotomy. A subtle parastomal hernia may be appreciated by asking the patient to perform a Valsalva manoeuvre or raise the head off the bed. In the acute hospital setting, overlying skin changes should be assessed, and the stoma should be digitated.

Although a diagnosis can be made on clinical assessment, cross-sectional imaging with computed tomography (CT) or (in case of a specific indication defined by a clinician) magnetic resonance imaging (MRI) offers valuable information. In morbidly obese patients, these modalities may be the only way to make the diagnosis. Imaging also gives insight into the size of the defect, hernia contents, radiological anatomy, and quality of the abdominal wall musculature. It can also detect and assess any other concomitant intra-abdominal disease radiological appearances.

6. Classification

The European Hernia Society's (EHS) classification of parastomal hernias is based on hernia size, whether there is a concomitant incisional hernia and if the occurrence is a primary parastomal hernia or recurrence [19]. It is summarised in **Table 1**.

Classification	Description	Management principles
Type 1	≤5 cm without concomitant incisional hernia	Sugarbaker repair, open or MIS; keyhole or "sandwich" technique.
Type 2	≤5 cm with concomitant incisional hernia	Combined posterior compartment separation with Sugarbaker or keyhole repair.
Type 3	>5 cm without concomitant incisional hernia	Open/MIS Sugarbaker repair, keyhole technique or "sandwich." If hernia defect is very large, it may require a combined posterior compartment separation and/or relocation of stoma with consideration for STORRM and reinforcing the closure of the old ostomy site with mesh.
Type 4	>5 cm with concomitant incisional hernia	Combined posterior component separation with Sugarbaker or keyhole repair. If the hernia site is large and relocation of the stoma is planned, consider STORRM and reinforcing the closure of the old ostomy site with mesh.

P = Primary parastomal hernia.
R = Recurrent parastomal hernia.
MIS = Minimally invasive surgery. STORRM = Stapled Transabdominal Ostomy Reinforcement with Retromuscular Mesh.

Table 1.
European Hernia Society classification of parastomal hernia and its current management principles.

Parastomal hernia repair, by its nature, involves surgery of an ostomy producing bowel or urinary contents. The Modified Ventral Hernia Working Group (VHWG) would, therefore, classify any parastomal repair as a Grade 3, contaminated procedure, which carries a high risk of surgical site infection (SSI) of 46% [20]. Consequently, the high risk of SSI impacts the decision of mesh choice. In a contaminated field, a biological mesh may be favourable, but evidence for the use of biological vs. permanent mesh in parastomal hernia repair is weak. The European Hernia Society makes no recommendation regarding the type of mesh used [21]. The limited literature does not report any difference in postoperative complications for parastomal hernia repair using a biological or synthetic mesh [22–24].

7. Guidelines

Guidelines for parastomal hernia prevention and management have been published by the European Hernia Society (EHS) and the American Society of Colon and Rectal Surgeons (ASCRS) [21, 25]. Recommendation statements are graded on the strength of the recommendation and the strength of the assessed evidence. A summary of guidelines pertaining to parastomal hernia is provided in **Table 2**.

The main difference between the two guidelines is that the EHS recommends using a prophylactic mesh when creating an end colostomy, whilst the ASCRS does not recommend this based on the available evidence. The ASCRC suggests that tunnelling an end colostomy may reduce the risk of parastomal hernia formation, whilst the EHS makes no recommendation.

Item	Recommendation	Strength
European Hernia Society, 2018		
1	Clinical examination in supine/erect position and using the Valsalva manoeuvre is necessary for the diagnosis of parastomal hernia, whereas CT scan or ultrasonography may be performed in uncertain cases.	Weak
2	No recommendation can be made on the policy of watchful waiting for patients with a non-incarcerated parastomal hernia.	NA
3	No recommendation can be made in preference of stoma construction through the extraperitoneal over the transperitoneal route.	NA
4	No recommendation can be made in preference of stoma construction at a lateral pararectus location over a transrectus location.	NA
5	We suggest keeping the size of the fascial aperture as small as possible to allow passage of the intestine through the abdominal wall without causing ischaemia.	Weak
6	It is recommended to use a prophylactic synthetic non-absorbable mesh when constructing an elective permanent end colostomy to reduce the parastomal hernia rate.	Strong
7	No recommendation to use a prophylactic mesh can be made for ileostomies or ileal conduit stomas, nor for the use of synthetic absorbable or biological meshes.	NA
8	It is recommended not to perform a suture repair for elective parastomal hernia surgery because of a high risk of recurrence.	Strong
9	No recommendation can be made in favour of laparoscopic or open parastomal hernia repair with a mesh in elective surgery.	NA
10	No recommendation can be made in favour of any open parastomal hernia repair with mesh.	NA
11	For laparoscopic parastomal hernia repair, a mesh without a hole is suggested in preference to a keyhole mesh.	Weak
12	No recommendation can be made on the use of specific mesh material for parastomal hernia repair.	NA
American Society of Colon and Rectum Surgeons, 2022		
1	Potential ostomy sites should be marked preoperatively by a trained provider.	Strong
2	The routine use of prophylactic mesh to prevent parastomal hernia at the time of ostomy creation is not recommended.	Weak
3	Extraperitoneal tunnelling of an end colostomy may decrease the risk of parastomal hernia.	Weak
4	Parastomal hernia repair should typically utilise mesh reinforcement.	Strong
5	Minimally invasive parastomal hernia repair may be performed in selected patients.	Strong

Table 2.
Summary of the European Hernia Society and the American Society of Colon and Rectum Surgeons guidelines.

8. Management

8.1 Stoma reversal

When encountering a patient with a parastomal hernia in an outpatient clinic, an initial consideration is the history of the stoma and whether the ostomy can be reversed in order to improve or restore the quality of life of the patient. In those patients with potential for reversal, consideration must be given to the suitability for major abdominal surgery, risks of intestinal anastomosis formation, and patient wishes. If a suitable option, reversal is a definitive management of a parastomal hernia. Closure of the defect in the abdominal wall can be reinforced with the placement of a mesh.

8.2 Watchful waiting

A process of watchful waiting may be adopted in patients who are either averse to surgical intervention or have only mild symptoms. However, considerations for this method need to be discussed with the patient thoroughly, as there is potential for the hernia to increase in size over time and for incarceration to occur. Also, during the discussion, it must be mentioned that an emergency repair will carry increased postoperative morbidity to the patient. Furthermore, with a prolonged timeframe of watchful waiting, the patient may develop concurrent medical problems, which would make surgery at a later date more high risk. Although it is common practice, there is no high-level published evidence base for watchful waiting for a parastomal hernia, as shown in **Table 2** [21].

8.3 Emergency vs. elective surgery

In the emergency setting, the primary focus is on releasing incarcerated or obstructed bowel, ensuring the patient is safe from the emergency. Repair of the parastomal hernia is then the second surgical priority.

Other considerations in the emergency general surgery setting include the patient's overall health and suitability for a longer general anaesthetic and operation, potentially ischaemic, necrotic, or perforated bowel requiring resection, and the impact of a contaminated wound on mesh choice and wound healing.

8.4 Primary suture repair

It is the most straightforward and least morbid operative approach for repairing a parastomal hernia. The essence of this operation is a peri-stomal incision, the hernia sac exposure from surrounding tissue, and reduction of the viable hernia contents onto the free peritoneal cavity. The musculofascial defect of the abdominal wall is then closed with absorbable or non-absorbable sutures. Due to the high recurrence rates, 46–100% [21, 26], this method is reserved only for emergency cases and where the patient has limited life expectancy or extensive medical co-morbidities that mean a more complex operation is unsuitable.

8.5 Stoma relocation

Relocating the stoma to another site of the abdominal wall may be beneficial if the original site of the stoma and the parastomal hernia were causing problems applying stoma appliances or discomfort with clothing. However, as a technique for parastomal hernia treatment, it comes with multiple pitfalls. Often, a relocation of the ostomy will require laparotomy, and there is a substantial risk of repeat herniation across the abdominal wall at the old stoma site (52%) [27], new stoma location (48%) [28], and midline laparotomy area (20%) [29]. If stoma relocation is performed, closure of the old stoma site should be reinforced with mesh [30].

Stapled Transabdominal Ostomy Reinforcement with Retro-muscular Mesh (STORRM) has been trialled to reduce the parastomal hernia rates at the new stoma site when relocating stomas [31]. This surgical technique can be briefly described as follows: the abdomen is opened by middle laparotomy, posterior component separation with transversus abdominis release is completed, a mesh is placed in the retro-muscular space, and the stoma is matured using a circle stapling device. Initial reports of 12 cases showed no recurrence at 1 year [31].

8.6 Mesh parastomal hernia repairs

8.6.1 Sugarbaker repair and keyhole technique

First described in 1985, the Sugarbaker repair involves the reduction of the hernia sac into the abdomen and lateralising the stoma using intraperitoneal mesh [32]. The keyhole technique similarly uses an intraperitoneal mesh, but instead of lateralising the bowel, an opening is created in the centre of the mesh, and the bowel passes through this and then the abdominal wall in a linear manner.

The keyhole technique has been modified into a retro-muscular mesh placement, whereby the stoma is taken down and then re-matured through the abdominal wall, incorporating the mesh [33]. This technique has the advantage of not requiring extra bowel length for the necessary lateralisation in a Sugarbaker repair.

Meta-analysis has not demonstrated convincing evidence for the efficacy of one repair over the other [34, 35]. The Sugarbaker and keyhole techniques have been combined into a "sandwich technique" [36]. Recently, a modification of the Sugarbaker technique has been described by Pauli where a posterior component separation with transversus abdominis release is combined with mesh reinforcement of a modified Sugarbaker in the retro-muscular space; the stoma is left in situ [37]. There was an 11% recurrence rate at one institute at 13 months following this repair; 8% of patients experienced mesh erosion.

8.6.2 Concomitant midline hernia

Where there is a concomitant midline hernia, any operative plan must include dealing with both hernias. To achieve this, a posterior compartment separation with ipsilateral or bilateral transversus abdominis release is performed alongside a parastomal hernia repair technique. As discussed above, if the stoma is to be left in situ and there is enough bowel length for lateralisation, a Pauli repair is a method of achieving this. Otherwise, the abdominal wall release can be combined with a standard Sugarbaker or keyhole-type repair. Where the stoma is being relocated, the compartment separation can be combined with a STORRM technique or the new stoma reinforced with mesh.

8.6.3 Minimally invasive approach

Sugarbaker and keyhole techniques have been modified to be performed both laparoscopically and robotically. The advantages of minimally invasive abdominal surgery are well established. A recent meta-analysis of laparoscopic data for Sugarbaker and keyhole techniques reported the incidence of postoperative complications as 31.3% versus 27.6%, respectively, and recurrence of 24.1% versus 9% [38]. Further meta-analysis has shown advantages in postoperative complications and recurrence in laparoscopic Sugarbaker and keyhole procedures compared with open

Author, year	Surgical approach	Technique	References
Yang, 2017	Laparoscopic	Keyhole, Sugarbaker, "Sandwich"	[43]
Rege, 2019	Laparoscopic	Modified Sugarbaker	[44]
Bellido-Luque, 2023	Laparoscopic	Modified Sugarbaker	[45]
Maciel, 2019	Robotic	Retro-rectus repair	[46]
Morrell, 2020	Robotic	Modified retromuscular Sugarbaker (Pauli)	[47]
Bloemendaal, 2023	Robotic	Retromuscular parastomal hernia repair (Pauli)	[48]
Barranquero, 2024	Robotic	Modified retromuscular Sugarbaker (Pauli)	[49]
Lambrecht, 2024	Robotic	Pauli repair	[50]

Table 3.
Minimal invasive surgical approaches and techniques, 2017–2024.

approaches. Both repair techniques laparoscopically had comparable outcomes [39]. Robotic data is still in its infancy but offers promising results, with recurrence following Sugarbaker repair being reported between 5.8% and 6.7% at 14 months [40–42].

The decision to attempt a minimally invasive parastomal hernia repair depends on the surgeon's experience, skills, and the nature of the parastomal hernia. Any decision should be made jointly with the patient after consultation and a period of reflection (**Table 3**).

9. Prevention of parastomal hernia

9.1 Stoma site location

The current consensus is to create stomas through the rectus sheaths and the middle of the rectus abdominus muscle, with a historic paper showing a reduced incidence of parastomal hernia compared with a lateral pararectus approach (3% vs. 22%) [51]. However, a Cochrane review of 761 patients across nine studies found no significant difference between a transrectus or lateral pararectus approach (relative risk: 1.29 [0.79–2.1]) [52]. However, this review was limited by the heterogeneity and low quality of the papers included.

9.2 Rectus muscle sheath incision

A classic surgical description of a stoma formation is to make a cruciate incision in the rectus sheaths to allow the passage of the bowel. It had been hypothesised that the shape of the incision—cruciate versus circular—may impact parastomal hernia development due to differing points of weakness created within the sheath. A randomised control trial published in 2021 did not find any difference in stoma complications, including parastomal hernia, when a cruciate or circular incision was made to the sheath.

9.3 Prophylactic mesh

The EHS recommends using a prophylactic synthetic, non-absorbable mesh when creating an elective permanent end colostomy to reduce the risk of parastomal hernia [21, 25]. This recommendation is supported by meta-analysis data showing a significant reduction in the incidence of parastomal hernia when prophylactic mesh was used (odds ratio: 0.60 [0.46–0.80]) [53]. However, the literature on prophylactic mesh is inconclusive, with a more recent meta-analysis presenting contradictory findings that the incidence of parastomal hernia was not reduced when a prophylactic mesh was placed (relative risk: 0.68 [0.46–1.02]) [54]. A further long-term study showed, at 5 years of follow-up, no difference in parastomal hernia rates, with prophylactic mesh delaying the onset of parastomal hernia without a significant difference in morbidity, mortality, or quality of life [6].

The concern regarding mesh infections, erosion, or other stoma complications related to placing prophylactic mesh in the retro-muscular plane has been alleviated. Multiple review articles report no significant increase in postoperative complications from mesh placement [55–57]. Also, the advent of a new generation of multi-layer biological meshes reinforced by a polymer may strengthen the concept of preventing parastomal hernia repair.

10. Conclusions

The incidence of parastomal hernia is high, particularly in end colostomies performed in emergency settings. In the elective setting, repair should be performed by a surgeon with a specialist interest. Depending on the hernia size and concomitant incisional hernia, a mesh-based repair, open or minimally invasive, should be performed with or without component separation surgery.

Conflict of interest

The authors declare no conflict of interest.

Author details

Adam Daniel Gerrard* and Raimundas Lunevicius
Liverpool University Hospitals NHS Foundation Trust, Aintree Hospital, Liverpool, UK

*Address all correspondence to: adamgerrard@doctors.org.uk

References

[1] Hardy KJ. Evolution of the stoma. Australian and New Zealand Journal of Surgery. 1989;**59**(1):71-77

[2] Colostomy UK. What is a Stoma? 2024. Available from: https://www.colostomyuk.org/information/what-is-a-stoma/

[3] Wasserman MA, MF MG. Preoperative considerations for the ostomate. Clinics in Colon and Rectal Surgery. 2017;**30**(3):157-161

[4] Carne P, Robertson G, Frizelle F. Parastomal hernia. The British Journal of Surgery. 2003;**90**(7):784-793

[5] Park J, Rivard SJ, Maguire L, Varlamos C, Duby A, Hendren S. Parastomal hernia rates and exercise after ostomy surgery. Diseases of the Colon & Rectum. 2023;**66**(6):823-830

[6] Brandsma HT, Hansson BM, Aufenacker TJ, de Jong N, Engelenburg KCV, Mahabier C, et al. Prophylactic mesh placement during formation of an end-colostomy: Long-term randomized controlled trial on effectiveness and safety. Annals of Surgery. 2023;**278**(3):e440-e6

[7] Robertson I, Leung E, Hughes D, Spiers M, Donnelly L, Mackenzie I, et al. Prospective analysis of stoma-related complications. Colorectal Disease. 2005;7(3):279-285

[8] Ripoche J, Basurko C, Fabbro-Perray P, Prudhomme M. Parastomal hernia. A study of the French federation of ostomy patients. Journal of Visceral Surgery. 2011;**148**(6):e435-e441

[9] Andersen RM, Klausen TW, Danielsen AK, Vinther A, Gögenur I, Thomsen T. Incidence and risk factors for parastomal bulging in patients with ileostomy or colostomy: A register-based study using data from the Danish Stoma Database Capital Region. Colorectal Disease. 2018;**20**(4):331-340

[10] Sohn YJ, Moon SM, Shin US, Jee SH. Incidence and risk factors of parastomal hernia. Journal of the Korean Society of Coloproctology. 2012;**28**(5):241-246

[11] Hong SY, Oh SY, Lee JH, Kim DY, Suh KW. Risk factors for parastomal hernia: Based on radiological definition. Journal of the Korean Surgical Society. 2013;**84**(1):43-47

[12] Niu N, Du S, Yang D, Zhang L, Wu B, Zhi X, et al. Risk factors for the development of a parastomal hernia in patients with enterostomy: A systematic review and meta-analysis. International Journal of Colorectal Disease. 2022;**37**(3):507-519

[13] Manole TE, Daniel I, Alexandra B, Dan PN, Andronic O. Risk factors for the development of parastomal hernia: A narrative review. Saudi Journal of Medicine & Medical Sciences. 2023;**11**(3):187-192

[14] Temple B, Farley T, Popik K, Ewanyshyn C, Beyer E, Dufault B. Prevalence of parastomal hernia and factors associated with its development. Journal of Wound, Ostomy, and Continence Nursing. 2016;**43**(5):489-493

[15] Zhao F, Chen F, Yuan X, Liu Y, Chen J. Decreased collagen type III synthesis in skin fibroblasts is associated with parastomal hernia following colostomy. International Journal of Molecular Medicine. Nov 2019;**44**(5):1609-1618

[16] Pu YW, Yang XD, Gong W, Xing CG. Etiological analysis of parastomal hernia by computed tomography examination. Wideochirurgia I Inne Techniki Maloinwazyjne. 2019;**14**(3):387-393

[17] Tivenius M, Näsvall P, Sandblom G. Parastomal hernias causing symptoms or requiring surgical repair after colorectal cancer surgery-a national population-based cohort study. International Journal of Colorectal Disease. 2019;**34**(7):1267-1272

[18] Zelga P, Kluska P, Zelga M, Piasecka-Zelga J, Dziki A. Patient-related factors associated with stoma and peristomal complications following fecal ostomy surgery: A scoping review. Journal of Wound, Ostomy, and Continence Nursing. 2021;**48**(5): 415-430

[19] Śmietański M, Szczepkowski M, Alexandre JA, Berger D, Bury K, Conze J, et al. European Hernia Society classification of parastomal hernias. Hernia. 2014;**18**(1):1-6

[20] Kanters AE, Krpata DM, Blatnik JA, Novitsky YM, Rosen MJ. Modified hernia grading scale to stratify surgical site occurrence after open ventral hernia repairs. Journal of the American College of Surgeons. 2012;**215**(6):787-793

[21] Antoniou SA, Agresta F, Garcia Alamino JM, Berger D, Berrevoet F, Brandsma HT, et al. European Hernia Society guidelines on prevention and treatment of parastomal hernias. Hernia. 2018;**22**(1):183-198

[22] Miller BT, Krpata DM, Petro CC, Beffa LRA, Carbonell AM, Warren JA, et al. Biologic vs synthetic mesh for parastomal hernia repair: Post hoc analysis of a multicenter randomized controlled trial. Journal of the American College of Surgeons. 2022;**235**(3):401-409

[23] Carbonell AM, Criss CN, Cobb WS, Novitsky YW, Rosen MJ. Outcomes of synthetic mesh in contaminated ventral hernia repairs. Journal of the American College of Surgeons. 2013;**217**(6):991-998

[24] Slater NJ, Hansson BM, Buyne OR, Hendriks T, Bleichrodt RP. Repair of parastomal hernias with biologic grafts: A systematic review. Journal of Gastrointestinal Surgery. 2011;**15**(7):1252-1258

[25] Davis BR, Valente MA, Goldberg JE, Lightner AL, Feingold DL, Paquette IM. The American Society of colon and rectal surgeons clinical practice guidelines for ostomy surgery. Diseases of the Colon and Rectum. 2022;**65**(10):1173-1190

[26] Roussel B, Mulieri G, Gauzolino R, Danion J, De Wailly P, Faure JP. Parastomal hernia. Journal of Visceral Surgery. 2012;**149**(5 Suppl):e15-e19

[27] Rubin MS, Schoetz DJ Jr, Matthews JB, Parastomal hernia. Is stoma relocation superior to fascial repair? Archives of Surgery. 1994;**129**(4):413-418; discussion 8-9

[28] Riansuwan W, Hull TL, Millan MM, Hammel JP. Surgery of recurrent parastomal hernia: Direct repair or relocation? Colorectal Disease. 2010;**12**(7):681-686

[29] Hu A, Pauli EM. Management of parastomal hernias. Seminars in Colon and Rectal Surgery. 2023;**34**(2):100956

[30] Bhangu A, Nepogodiev D, Ives N, Magill L, Glasbey J, Forde C, et al. Prophylactic biological mesh reinforcement versus standard closure of stoma site (ROCSS): A multicentre, randomised controlled trial. The Lancet. 2020;**395**(10222):417-426

[31] Majumder A, Orenstein SB, Miller HJ, Novitsky YW. Stapled Transabdominal Ostomy Reinforcement with retromuscular mesh (STORRM): Technical details and early outcomes of a novel approach for retromuscular repair of parastomal hernias. The American Journal of Surgery. 2018;**215**(1):82-87

[32] Sugarbaker PH. Peritoneal approach to prosthetic mesh repair of paraostomy hernias. Annals of Surgery. 1985;**201**(3):344-346

[33] Raigani S, Criss CN, Petro CC, Prabhu AS, Novitsky YW, Rosen MJ. Single-center experience with parastomal hernia repair using retromuscular mesh placement. Journal of Gastrointestinal Surgery. 2014;**18**(9):1673-1677

[34] Fleming AM, Phillips AL, Drake JA, Gross MG, Yakoub D, Monroe J, et al. Sugarbaker versus keyhole repair for parastomal hernia: A systematic review and meta-analysis of comparative studies. Journal of Gastrointestinal Surgery. 2023;**27**(3):573-584

[35] Mäkäräinen-Uhlbäck E, Vironen J, Vaarala M, Nordström P, Välikoski A, Kössi J, et al. Keyhole versus Sugarbaker techniques in parastomal hernia repair following ileal conduit urinary diversion: A retrospective nationwide cohort study. BMC Surgery. 2021;**21**(1):231

[36] Berger D, Bientzle M. Laparoscopic repair of parastomal hernias: A single surgeon's experience in 66 patients. Diseases of the Colon and Rectum. 2007;**50**(10):1668-1673

[37] Pauli EM, Juza RM, Winder JS. How I do it: Novel parastomal herniorrhaphy utilizing transversus abdominis release. Hernia. 2016;**20**(4):547-552

[38] Kritharides N, Papaconstantinou D, Kykalos S, Machairas N, Schizas D, Nikiteas NI, et al. Laparoscopic parastomal hernia repair: Keyhole, Sugarbaker, sandwich, or hybrid technique with 3D mesh? An updated systematic review and meta-analysis. Langenbeck's Archives of Surgery. 2023;**408**(1):448

[39] Sarno G, Iacone B, Tedesco A, Gargiulo A, Ranieri A, Giordano A, et al. End-colostomy parastomal hernia repair: A systematic review on laparoscopic and robotic approaches. Hernia. 2024;**28**(3):723-743

[40] Ferrari D, Violante T, Gomaa IA, Cima RR. Robotic modified Sugarbaker technique for parastomal hernia repair: A standardized approach. Updates in Surgery. 2024;**76**(3):1115-1119

[41] Ayuso SA, Shao JM, Deerenberg EB, Elhage SA, George MB, Heniford BT, et al. Robotic Sugarbaker parastomal hernia repair: Technique and outcomes. Hernia. 2021;**25**(3):809-815

[42] Violante T, Ferrari D, Gomaa IA, Aboelmaaty SA, Behm KT, Cima RR. Robotic parastomal hernia repair: A single-center cohort study. Updates in Surgery. Nov 2024;**76**(7):2627-2634

[43] Yang X, He K, Hua R, Shen Q, Yao Q. Laparoscopic repair of parastomal hernia. Annals of Translational Medicine. 2017;**5**(3):45

[44] Rege S, Singh A, Rewatkar A, Murugan J, Menezes R, Surpam S, et al. Laparoscopic parastomal hernia repair: A modified technique of mesh placement in Sugarbaker procedure. Journal of Minimal Access Surgery. 2019;**15**(3):224-228

[45] Bellido-Luque J, Bellido-Luque A, Gomez-Rosado JC, Gomez-Menchero J, Suarez-Grau JM, Licardie E, et al. Full endoscopic minimally invasive

extraperitoneal modified Sugarbaker approach for para-colostomy hernia repair: Technical aspects and 2-year follow-up results of a prospective cohort. Colorectal Disease. 2023;**25**(10):2033-2042

[46] Maciel V, Mata W, Arevalo G, Zeichen M, Glass T. Robotic retro-rectus repair of parastomal hernias. Journal of Robotic Surgery. 2019;**13**(3):483-489

[47] Morrell DJ, Blatnik JA, Pauli EM. Robotic Parastomal Hernia Repair: Modified Retromuscular Sugarbaker. In: Kudsi O, editor. Robotic Hernia Surgery. Cham: Springer; 2020

[48] Bloemendaal ALA. Robotic retromuscular (recurrent) parastomal hernia repair (r-Pauli-repair) with synthetically reinforced biological mesh; technique, early experience, and short-term follow-up. Journal of Abdominal Wall Surgery. 2023;**2**:12059

[49] Barranquero AG, Maestre González Y, Gas Ruiz C, Sadurni Gracia M, Olsina Kissler JJ, Villalobos MR. Early outcomes of robotic modified retromuscular Sugarbaker technique for end colostomy parastomal hernia repair. Hernia. 2024;**28**(6):2235-2243

[50] Lambrecht JR. Robotic Pauli repair of parastomal hernia. Surgical Endoscopy. 2024;**38**(10):6161-6168

[51] Sjödahl R, Anderberg B, Bolin T. Parastomal hernia in relation to site of the abdominal stoma. The British Journal of Surgery. 1988;**75**(4):339-341

[52] Hardt J, Meerpohl JJ, Metzendorf MI, Kienle P, Post S, Herrle F. Lateral pararectal versus transrectal stoma placement for prevention of parastomal herniation. Cochrane Database of Systematic Reviews. 2013;(11). Article No: CD009487

[53] McKechnie T, Lee J, Lee Y, Doumouras A, Amin N, Hong D, et al. Prophylactic mesh for prevention of parastomal hernia following end colostomy: An updated systematic review and meta-analysis of randomized controlled trials. Journal of Gastrointestinal Surgery. 2022;**26**(2):486-502

[54] Verdaguer-Tremolosa M, Garcia-Alamino JM, Rodrigues-Gonçalves V, Martínez-López MP, López-Cano M. Prophylactic mesh does not prevent parastomal hernia in long-term: Meta-analysis and trial sequential analysis. Surgery. 2024;**175**(2):441-450

[55] Shabbir J, Chaudhary BN, Dawson R. A systematic review on the use of prophylactic mesh during primary stoma formation to prevent parastomal hernia formation. Colorectal Disease. 2012;**14**(8):931-936

[56] Wijeyekoon SP, Gurusamy K, El-Gendy K, Chan CL. Prevention of parastomal herniation with biologic/composite prosthetic mesh: A systematic review and meta-analysis of randomized controlled trials. Journal of the American College of Surgeons. 2010;**211**(5):637-645

[57] Tam KW, Wei PL, Kuo LJ, Wu CH. Systematic review of the use of a mesh to prevent parastomal hernia. World Journal of Surgery. 2010;**34**(11):2723-2729

Chapter 5

Post-Herniorrhaphy Pain: A Frequent Complication in a Common Procedure

Mehmet Berksun Tutan

Abstract

Post-herniorrhaphy pain (PHP) is a prevalent and challenging complication following inguinal hernia repair, characterized by persistent pain lasting beyond 3 months. While most postoperative pain resolves within 6 to 8 weeks, PHP persists in a significant subset of patients, severely impacting their quality of life. This pain is primarily neuropathic, often resulting from intraoperative nerve injuries or secondary inflammatory processes, with key contributors including the ilioinguinal, iliohypogastric, genitofemoral, and lateral femoral cutaneous nerves. Additionally, mesh-related complications, such as nerve entrapment or chronic inflammation, play a critical role. Central sensitization further exacerbates PHP by amplifying pain signals, leading to heightened pain sensitivity and chronicity. Risk factors include younger age, preoperative pain, and severe acute postoperative pain. Diagnosis requires a detailed clinical evaluation and usually involves imaging or diagnostic nerve blocks. Management strategies range from pharmacologic therapies and nerve blocks to surgical interventions, including neurectomy and mesh revision. Preventive measures, such as meticulous nerve identification, optimal mesh selection, and effective perioperative pain management, are essential to reduce PHP incidence. As surgical techniques and technologies advance, a multidisciplinary approach to PHP can improve outcomes and enhance patient quality of life.

Keywords: inguinal hernia, post-operative pain, chronic complications, hernia surgery, post-operative inguinodynia

1. Introduction

The concept of hernia has been recognized since ancient times, with descriptions found in Egyptian, Greek, and Roman medical texts [1–3]. The term itself was first systematically used in medical literature during the Roman era, particularly by Celsus in the first century AD in his medical compendium De Medicina [3]. Celsus described various types of hernias and their treatments, including surgical techniques, making him one of the earliest physicians to use the term in a clinical context [3]. Later, the term was further formalized in medical lexicons during the Middle Ages and Renaissance as medical science developed [1, 2]. Thus, while the concept of hernia has existed for millennia, the coinage and consistent use of the term in medical literature can be traced back to Roman antiquity, around the first century AD.

IntechOpen

Historically, management of inguinal hernia was rudimentary and fraught with complications. These early approaches primarily involved compressive bandages or crude surgical attempts to reduce hernias [4]. The Renaissance and Enlightenment periods brought significant progress in anatomical understanding through works such as Vesalius [4]. During the eighteenth and nineteenth centuries, surgeons like Antonio Scarpa and Astley Cooper contributed critical insights into the anatomy of the inguinal region, including the description of the inguinal canal and the pathophysiology of hernias [5]. The modern era of inguinal hernia repair began in the late nineteenth century with the advent of antiseptic techniques and general anesthesia, which made surgery safer and more accessible. One of the most significant milestones was the development of the tension-based repair technique by Edoardo Bassini in 1887 [1]. In the mid-twentieth century, the introduction of tension-free repair revolutionized inguinal hernia surgery; Irving Lichtenstein's technique, described in the 1980s, involved the use of synthetic mesh to reinforce the posterior wall of the inguinal canal without creating tension on the tissues, and it is now the gold standard of hernia repair [1, 2, 5]. The late twentieth and early twenty-first centuries saw the emergence of minimally invasive techniques, including laparoscopic and robotic-assisted hernia repairs [6]. More recently, robotic-assisted surgery has refined minimally invasive hernia repair by providing enhanced visualization, greater precision, and improved ergonomics for the surgeon [6]. Inguinal hernia surgery continues to evolve with the integration of emerging technologies, but pain, both before and after surgery, is still a significant point of care in surgery.

Post-herniorrhaphy pain (PHP) is a chronic pain syndrome that persists for more than 3 months following the surgical repair of a hernia [7]. This condition is distinguished from acute postoperative pain and represents a significant deviation from the expected healing trajectory [8]. PHP is characterized by pain localized to the surgical site and may present as a burning, stabbing, or aching sensation [7]. In some cases, the pain radiates to adjacent regions, such as the groin or scrotum, and is often accompanied by sensory disturbances, including hypersensitivity, paresthesia, or numbness. The severity of PHP varies considerably, ranging from mild discomfort to severe debilitating pain that markedly impairs function and quality of life [8, 9].

2. Etiology and pathophysiology

Pain is a frequent postoperative outcome following herniorrhaphy, typically subsiding within approximately 2 months [10]. However, in some patients, the pain persists, with a subset developing moderate-to-severe pain that can significantly impair quality of life, including sexual function [11]. Persistent pain lasting beyond 3 months post-surgery, unassociated with other conditions such as seroma or hematoma, is commonly classified as post-herniorrhaphy neuralgia [12].

Chronic pain after groin hernia repair is relatively prevalent, though its reported incidence varies widely. Studies show that up to half of the patients report some level of residual groin pain at 1 year, while 15% experience moderate-to-severe pain that may be disabling [7, 10]. Studies indicate that chronic pain can occur in up to 36.7% of patients after herniorrhaphy, with the incidence of chronic pain varying widely in the literature, reported between 11% and 53% [7–9, 13–15]. In a large prospective study of 781 elective open hernia repairs, 16.5% of patients reported persistent pain at 6 months, which remained similar at 5 years (16.1%). However, moderate-to-severe pain was documented in only 1.2% at 6 months and 1.5% at 5 years [16, 17].

The mechanisms underlying post-herniorrhaphy pain are complex and multifactorial, encompassing both inflammatory and neuropathic processes [18]. Two main distinct mechanisms can result in a perception of pain following surgery. Acute postoperative pain is primarily driven by nociceptive and inflammatory responses, which typically diminish within 6 to 8 weeks [11]. In contrast, chronic neuropathic pain arises from abnormal nerve activity, often persisting even in the absence of ongoing inflammation [10, 11]. This pain is frequently linked to nerve injuries sustained during surgery, either directly or secondarily, due to complications like inflammation or entrapment. Thus, if post-herniorrhaphy groin pain persists for more than 8 weeks, it is most likely neuropathic in nature and can be due to primary or secondary nerve injuries [14, 19].

In chronic pain, neuropathic mechanisms play a central role, often stemming from nerve injuries sustained during surgery. These injuries frequently involve the ilioinguinal, iliohypogastric, or genitofemoral nerves, which can lead to persistent sensory dysfunction and neuropathic pain syndromes [18]. Such injuries typically occur intraoperatively and may involve complete or partial nerve transection, potentially resulting in neuroma formation. Additional causes of nerve damage include mechanical manipulation during surgery, such as stretching, crushing, or cautery injury [20, 21]. Nerve entrapment by sutures, staples, or implanted mesh is another well-documented factor contributing to prolonged pain [21, 22].

The cutaneous nerves of the lower abdomen and groin most commonly implicated in persistent post-herniorrhaphy pain include the ilioinguinal, iliohypogastric, genitofemoral, and lateral femoral cutaneous nerves [23]. These nerves originate from the lumbar plexus and provide sensory innervation to the groin, upper hip, and thigh regions [24]. During open hernia repair, the iliohypogastric, ilioinguinal, and genital branch of the genitofemoral nerves are frequently encountered. At the same time, laparoscopic or preperitoneal approaches may expose the lateral femoral cutaneous nerve, the femoral branch of the genitofemoral nerve, and, occasionally, the femoral nerve [2, 24]. Although injury to the lateral femoral cutaneous nerve is less common, it can occur when the inguinal ligament and the lateral fibers of the internal oblique aponeurosis are divided [24]. Injury or entrapment of any of these nerves can lead to chronic postoperative pain [21, 24].

Inflammatory and musculoskeletal factors also play a significant role in persistent pain. Chronic inflammatory reactions to foreign materials, such as mesh, and mechanical irritation of adjacent tissues are common causes of PHP [20]. Secondary nerve injuries may result from inflammation adjacent to the nerve, most frequently caused by mesh placement [20, 22]. Contact between peripheral nerves and polypropylene mesh can induce myelin sheath degeneration, edema, and fibrosis, contributing to nerve damage [21, 22]. Additionally, improper positioning or folding of the mesh may entrap nerves, exacerbating pain symptoms [25, 26].

A phenomenon known as "central sensitization" can further perpetuate post-herniorrhaphy pain by amplifying pain signals, leading to chronic pain even after the resolution of the initial nociceptive injury [27]. This phenomenon is characterized by heightened responsiveness of nociceptive neurons in the central nervous system to both normal and subthreshold inputs. The resulting increased pain sensitivity facilitates the transition from acute to chronic pain and manifests as hyperalgesia (exaggerated pain response to stimuli) or allodynia (pain triggered by ordinarily non-painful stimuli) [27, 28]. These mechanisms contribute to the persistence of pain long after the surgical site has healed, complicating management and recovery [29, 30].

3. Risk factors

Persistent pain after groin hernia repair is influenced by various factors, such as patient demographics, preoperative conditions, surgical techniques, and postoperative complications [7, 8, 11, 17]. Key risk factors include younger age, preoperative pain, severe acute postoperative pain, a surgical interval of less than 3 years from a previous operation, and the presence of postoperative complications [7, 11]. Also, sensory disorders, female gender, recurrent hernia repair, damage to the iliohypogastric nerve, and the use of an anterior surgical approach are some of the reasons [31–33].

Younger age has consistently emerged as a critical risk factor, with studies indicating that patients under the age of 40 are far more likely to report chronic pain compared to older populations [34]. A study involving patients undergoing inguinal hernia surgery reported a persistent pain prevalence of 58% in individuals under 40, compared to 14% in those over 60 [7]. This disparity may be caused by increased physical demands and occupational stress associated with younger age groups, which could amplify postoperative discomfort and interfere with recovery [34]. Additionally, younger individuals may have heightened pain sensitivity, possibly due to more active nociceptive pathways or differing psychological responses to pain [34].

Preexisting pain in the inguinal region before surgery further predisposes patients to the development of persistent pain after hernia repair [11]. This phenomenon has been observed in other surgical contexts, such as amputation, thoracotomy, and breast surgery, where preoperative neuropathic or inflammatory pain sensitizes neural pathways [7, 11, 32]. Prospective studies in hernia repair report that patients with preoperative groin pain are significantly more likely to experience chronic pain both at 6 months and 5 years postoperatively [17].

Hernia size and class are regarded as significant factors influencing postoperative pain outcomes. In a study by Hoffmann et al. [35], hernias smaller than 1.5 cm were associated with a greater likelihood of persistent pain than larger hernias sized between 1.5 and 3 cm. Although the precise etiology remains unclear, it has been hypothesized that differing patient expectations may contribute to this observation [35].

Surgical technique has been identified as another critical determinant of postoperative pain [35, 36]. Open anterior approaches have been shown to carry a higher risk of chronic pain compared to laparoscopic or robotic procedures, where a posterior approach is utilized [36]. Additionally, the recurrence of hernias and surgical intervals of less than 3 years from a prior operation has been associated with an exacerbated risk of post-herniorrhaphy pain, likely attributable to increased scar tissue, altered anatomy, and heightened nerve sensitivity [11].

The severity of acute postoperative pain is widely recognized as a predictor of chronic pain development [11, 37]. Severe early postoperative pain has been implicated in the process of central sensitization, whereby the nervous system becomes hyperresponsive, perpetuating pain long after the original surgical insult has resolved [18, 34]. Postoperative complications, including hematomas, infections, and hernia recurrence, are understood to further compound this risk by prolonging tissue inflammation, impairing healing, and increasing neural irritation [35, 37].

Biological and psychosocial factors have also been observed to contribute to variability in pain outcomes. Female sex has been consistently associated with a higher prevalence of chronic postoperative pain, potentially due to hormonal influences, heightened nociceptive sensitivity, and differences in pain processing mechanisms [37–39]. Additional risk factors specific to women include a high body mass index, advanced American Society of Anesthesiologists (ASA) classification, and the presence of femoral hernias [39]. Interestingly, the mode of surgery (elective versus emergency) and specific surgical methods have not been shown to influence pain outcomes in female patients significantly [39]. Beyond biological factors, psychological aspects, including anxiety, depression, and chronic stress, have been implicated in shaping the pain experience [38]. These factors are thought to influence pain perception, coping mechanisms, and responses to analgesic therapies, further complicating the management of persistent pain [38].

4. Diagnosis and assessment

The diagnosis of post-herniorrhaphy pain requires a meticulous clinical evaluation, as it presents with persistent groin pain lasting beyond 6 to 8 weeks following inguinal hernia repair. This condition, distinct from typical acute postoperative pain, is predominantly neuropathic in nature, often accompanied by sensory changes and radiating pain along affected nerve pathways [12]. While the diagnosis is primarily clinical, imaging studies and advanced diagnostic techniques are essential in confirming the underlying cause and ruling out alternative explanations for the pain [10, 11].

A thorough clinical assessment is essential to identify key features of PHP. Pain localized to the surgical site and radiating along the distribution of the ilioinguinal, iliohypogastric, or genitofemoral nerves is a hallmark of the condition [10, 11]. Patients often describe the pain as burning, stabbing, or pricking, with specific triggers such as physical activity, palpation of the incision site, or even routine actions like coughing and breathing [26]. In many cases, this neuropathic pain is accompanied by sensory changes, including hyperesthesia, numbness, or paresthesia in the groin region [10]. Men may report additional symptoms, such as pain during ejaculation, indicative of genitofemoral nerve involvement [36, 40]. These features help differentiate PHP from inflammatory pain, which typically subsides without significant sensory deficits over time [13].

The clinical assessment must include a detailed patient history and physical examination. The history should explore the timing and progression of pain, its onset relative to surgery, and whether it was continuous or developed after a pain-free interval. The type of hernia, surgical approach, and intraoperative findings are essential factors that may influence the risk of PHP [11]. Preoperative groin pain, particularly in cases of recurrent hernia repair or prior abdominal surgeries, predisposes patients to chronic postoperative pain and should be carefully documented [32, 37]. Additionally, reports of acute postoperative complications, such as hematoma, mesh-related inflammation, or infection, should be noted, as these factors may exacerbate pain syndromes [34]. During the physical examination, specific attention should be paid to the distribution of pain and any sensory abnormalities in the groin. Reproduction of pain through palpation, particularly over the surgical site or the course of the affected nerves, supports a neuropathic origin [11, 18]. Tenderness near the pubic tubercle or anterior superior iliac spine may indicate nerve entrapment or mesh-induced irritation [22]. In some cases, pain may radiate to the upper thigh, scrotum, or labia, further highlighting the involvement of sensory nerves supplying these regions [22, 25].

Diagnostic imaging can complement the clinical evaluation, particularly when structural complications or recurrent hernia are suspected [20]. Modalities such as ultrasound, computed tomography (CT), and magnetic resonance imaging (MRI) are valuable in identifying non-neuropathic causes of pain, including mesh displacement, seromas, or fluid collections [20]. Among these, MRI, particularly with neurography, offers superior sensitivity in detecting nerve-related abnormalities, such as thickening, neuromas, or entrapment [41]. Although imaging is not always diagnostic for PHP, it is essential for ruling out alternative explanations that might necessitate surgical intervention, such as osteitis pubis or recurrent hernia [12].

Nerve blocks serve both diagnostic and therapeutic purposes in PHP [11]. The temporary relief of pain following the injection of a local anesthetic supports a diagnosis of nerve-related pain [11]. However, a negative response does not exclude PHP, as the presence of fibrosis or mesh-related inflammation may limit the spread of the anesthetic [11, 20, 25]. Advanced techniques, such as MR neurography, allow for more precise localization of nerve injuries, offering a potential tool for guiding targeted interventions [20, 41].

5. Management and treatment strategies

Effective management of post-herniorrhaphy pain requires a multimodal approach that addresses both the neuropathic and inflammatory components of the condition. Initial treatment strategies often include conservative measures, such as pharmacologic therapy with nonsteroidal anti-inflammatory drugs (NSAIDs) and analgesics. For most patients, postoperative groin pain resolves within 6 to 8 weeks [11]. However, in cases where pain persists beyond 3 months and is refractory to standard therapies, targeted interventions are necessary [42].

Nerve blocks are a cornerstone of PHP management, particularly for patients with confirmed neuropathic pain [42]. Performed by a pain specialist or surgeon familiar with the technique, these procedures involve the injection of a local anesthetic, often combined with a corticosteroid, around the affected nerve [43]. This approach not only alleviates pain but also provides diagnostic confirmation of nerve involvement [43]. Repeated injections may be administered for patients who achieve transient relief from nerve blocks, potentially breaking the pain cycle and leading to sustained improvement [42]. However, in cases where pain recurs after repeated nerve blocks, more definitive treatments such as nerve ablation or surgical neurectomy may be required [21].

Nerve ablation, using techniques such as radiofrequency ablation, cryoablation, or the injection of neurolytic agents like alcohol or phenol, offers a minimally invasive option for patients who respond to nerve blocks but experience recurrent pain [21]. This approach permanently destroys the offending nerve, reducing inflammation and preventing future irritation [44]. While outcomes for nerve ablation are generally favorable, recurrent pain due to nerve regeneration remains a potential limitation, necessitating further interventions in some cases [23].

Surgical neurectomy is the most definitive treatment for refractory PHP, with success rates reported as high as 90% in selected cases [23, 42]. Triple neurectomy, which involves excision of the ilioinguinal, iliohypogastric, and genital branch of the genitofemoral nerves, is particularly effective in cases of widespread nerve involvement [45, 46]. This procedure often requires concurrent mesh removal, as mesh-related fibrosis or entrapment commonly contributes to pain [47].

Mesh replacement in a different anatomical plane, such as the preperitoneal space, is recommended to minimize the risk of hernia recurrence while alleviating pain [46].

Emerging therapies, including nerve stimulation and the implantation of neuroprostheses, offer promising alternatives for patients with refractory pain or those who are poor candidates for surgical interventions [26]. While still experimental, these approaches may provide targeted pain relief by modulating nerve activity at the site of injury. Additionally, non-invasive adjuncts such as physical therapy, acupuncture, and topical analgesics can be considered, although their efficacy in chronic cases is limited [12, 23, 26].

6. Prevention

Preventing post-herniorrhaphy pain is a critical aspect of surgical planning and postoperative management. While the exact mechanisms leading to PHP are multifactorial and not entirely avoidable, several strategies have been identified to reduce the risk of chronic pain following inguinal hernia repair. These measures focus on optimizing surgical techniques, tailoring mesh use, and employing evidence-based perioperative interventions.

The meticulous identification and preservation of nerves during hernia repair are fundamental to reducing the risk of PHP [48]. Surgeons must carefully handle the ilioinguinal, iliohypogastric, and genitofemoral nerves to minimize the potential for intraoperative damage or entrapment. In cases where a nerve is suspected to be injured or at high risk of irritation due to the surgical field or mesh placement, prophylactic neurectomy may be considered [47, 48]. This approach has been supported by studies showing significant reductions in chronic pain among patients undergoing prophylactic ilioinguinal or iliohypogastric neurectomy during open hernia repair without an increase in sensory deficits or surgical complications [49].

The choice of surgical approach also impacts PHP risk [37]. Minimally invasive techniques, such as laparoscopic or robotic-assisted hernia repairs, are associated with lower rates of chronic pain compared to open anterior repairs [36]. This may be attributed to reduced tissue dissection, less nerve exposure, and superior visualization during mesh placement [36]. However, laparoscopic repairs are not without risk, as they may involve potential contact with the femoral nerve or lateral femoral cutaneous nerve in the preperitoneal space [33, 36]. Surgeons should weigh the benefits of each approach against individual patient factors to determine the most appropriate technique.

The use of mesh has become the standard of care for inguinal hernia repair due to its superior outcomes in preventing hernia recurrence [15]. However, mesh-associated complications, including inflammation, fibrosis, and nerve entrapment, are key contributors to PHP [15, 16]. Lightweight meshes, defined by a density of ≤ 50 g/m^2, have been associated with reduced rates of chronic pain and foreign body sensation compared to heavier meshes [50]. A meta-analysis comparing light versus heavy meshes demonstrated a statistically significant reduction in overall pain and discomfort with lightweight meshes while maintaining comparable hernia recurrence rates [51]. The use of self-gripping meshes, designed to eliminate the need for sutures or tacks, has shown mixed results, with some studies indicating no significant improvement in chronic pain or recurrence rates compared to standard suture-fixed meshes [52].

Mesh fixation methods also impact PHP risk [52]. Absorbable sutures for securing the mesh have demonstrated shorter durations and lower postoperative pain rates than nonabsorbable alternatives [53]. Similarly, fibrin glue has shown promise as a fixation method in both open and laparoscopic hernia repairs, significantly reducing postoperative pain while maintaining efficacy [54]. In contrast, cyanoacrylate glue and self-gripping mesh have not consistently demonstrated similar benefits, with conflicting results in randomized trials [12, 55]. Thus, the selection of fixation methods should be tailored to the patient's clinical presentation and the surgeon's expertise.

Anesthetic techniques employed during hernia repair can influence the incidence and severity of postoperative pain [46]. Local or regional anesthesia, such as spinal anesthesia, has been associated with lower postoperative pain levels than general anesthesia [30]. The continuous infusion of local anesthetics at the wound site has also shown efficacy in reducing early postoperative pain and may decrease the risk of chronic pain [30, 46].

Optimizing pain management during the perioperative period is essential for PHP prevention. Adequate control of acute postoperative pain reduces the risk of central sensitization, a phenomenon that can transition acute pain into chronic state [28, 30]. Multimodal analgesia, including NSAIDs, acetaminophen, and peripheral nerve blocks, is recommended to address pain through multiple mechanisms and minimize reliance on opioids [46, 48]. Emerging strategies, such as preoperative gabapentinoids or regional nerve blocks, have shown promise in reducing acute pain and improving long-term outcomes [43, 46, 48]. Prophylactic neurectomy, involving the routine removal of specific groin nerves during hernia repair, has been proposed as a preventive measure for PHP [49]. Meta-analyses have demonstrated that prophylactic ilioinguinal or iliohypogastric neurectomy during open hernia repair reduces the incidence of chronic pain, particularly in high-risk patients [47, 49]. However, this approach is not without trade-offs, as it may result in sensory deficits or dysesthesia in the nerve's distribution [49]. The decision to pursue prophylactic neurectomy should be individualized, considering patient preferences and surgical factors.

Emerging data highlight the potential benefits of preoperative optimization in reducing PHP risk. This includes addressing modifiable factors such as obesity, smoking, and poorly controlled diabetes, all of which are associated with increased postoperative complications [14, 35]. Intraoperative strategies to minimize tissue trauma, control bleeding, and prevent infection further contribute to improved pain outcomes [11]. Enhanced recovery after surgery protocols, emphasizing multimodal pain management, early mobilization, and patient education, can significantly reduce chronic pain after hernia repair [14].

By integrating these preventive strategies into surgical practice, the burden of PHP can be significantly reduced. Through a combination of advanced surgical techniques, judicious use of mesh and fixation methods, effective perioperative pain management, and patient-centered care, the incidence of this debilitating complication can be minimized, improving both surgical outcomes and quality of life for patients undergoing hernia repair.

7. Conclusion

Post-herniorrhaphy pain represents a significant challenge in the management of patients undergoing inguinal hernia repair. Despite advancements in surgical techniques, mesh materials, and pain management strategies, PHP remains a prevalent and debilitating complication, affecting a considerable proportion of patients. This chronic pain syndrome not only impacts physical function and quality of life but also places a burden on healthcare systems due to the need for long-term management.

DOI: http://dx.doi.org/10.5772/intechopen.1008766

The pathophysiology of PHP is complex and multifactorial, involving inflammatory, neuropathic, and central sensitization mechanisms. This complexity underscores the necessity for a thorough understanding of contributing factors, including patient-related risk factors, surgical techniques, and postoperative care. Comprehensive diagnosis requires a combination of clinical evaluation, advanced imaging, and selective diagnostic procedures, such as nerve blocks, to exclude alternative causes of groin pain and identify the underlying neuropathic component.

Management of PHP requires a multimodal and patient-centered approach. While pharmacologic therapies and nerve blocks remain the cornerstone of initial treatment, surgical interventions, including neurectomy and mesh revision, are invaluable for patients with refractory pain. Emerging techniques, such as nerve ablation, neuroprosthetic implants, and nerve stimulation, provide additional therapeutic avenues for those who do not respond to conventional measures.

Preventive strategies remain critical for reducing the incidence of PHP. Surgeons should aim to identify and preserve groin nerves during hernia repair and consider prophylactic neurectomy in high-risk patients. Mesh selection and fixation techniques, such as the use of lightweight meshes and absorbable sutures, can further minimize postoperative complications and chronic pain. By integrating preventive measures with effective diagnostic and therapeutic strategies, the burden of PHP can be significantly reduced, improving outcomes for affected patients.

In conclusion, while PHP remains a challenging complication of hernia repair, its impact can be mitigated through surgical precision, evidence-based management strategies, and ongoing advances in technology and research. By addressing the biological, technical, and patient-centered aspects of care, the burden of PHP can be reduced, improving outcomes and quality of life for patients undergoing hernia repair.

Acknowledgements

Thanks are due to my dearest family for their unwavering support through the most challenging times that befall us; to my wife and my little daughter, for always being the sunshine in the darkness, however dark it gets; and to Marica Novakovic for restoring my faith that kindness still exists.

Conflicts of interest

The author declares no conflict of interest.

Author details

Mehmet Berksun Tutan
Department of General Surgery, Alaca State Hospital, Çorum, Turkey

*Address all correspondence to: mbtutan@gmail.com

References

[1] Komorowski AL. History of the inguinal hernia repair. In: Silvestro C, editor. Inguinal Hernia. Rijeka: IntechOpen; 2014. Ch. 1

[2] Hori T, Yasukawa D. Fascinating history of groin hernias: Comprehensive recognition of anatomy, classic considerations for herniorrhaphy, and current controversies in hernioplasty. World Journal of Methodology. 2021;**11**(4):160-186

[3] Papavramidou NS, Christopoulou-Aletras H. Treatment of "hernia" in the writings of Celsus (first century AD). World Journal of Surgery. 2005;**29**(10):1343-1347

[4] Sachs M, Damm M, Encke A. Historical evolution of inguinal hernia repair. World Journal of Surgery. 1997;**21**(2):218-223

[5] Legutko J, Pach R, Solecki R, Matyja A, Kulig J. The history of treatment of groin hernia. Folia Medica Cracoviensia. 2008;**49**(1-2):57-74

[6] Lau WY. History of treatment of groin hernia. World Journal of Surgery. 2002;**26**(6):748-759

[7] Poobalan AS, Bruce J, Smith WC, King PM, Krukowski ZH, Chambers WA. A review of chronic pain after inguinal herniorrhaphy. The Clinical Journal of Pain. 2003;**19**(1):48-54

[8] Aasvang EK, Bay-Nielsen M, Kehlet H. Pain and functional impairment 6 years after inguinal herniorrhaphy. Hernia. 2006;**10**(4):316-321

[9] Kissin I, Gelman S. Chronic postsurgical pain: Still a neglected topic? Journal of Pain Research. 2012;**5**:473-489

[10] Bay-Nielsen M, Perkins FM, Kehlet H, Danish HD. Pain and functional impairment 1 year after inguinal herniorrhaphy: A nationwide questionnaire study. Annals of Surgery. 2001;**233**(1):1-7

[11] Kehlet H, Jensen TS, Woolf CJ. Persistent postsurgical pain: Risk factors and prevention. Lancet. 2006;**367**(9522):1618-1625

[12] Bonwich JB. Post-herniorrhaphy groin pain. In: Michael Rosen M, editor. UpToDate. Massachusetts: Wolters Kluwer; 2024

[13] Aasvang E, Kehlet H. Chronic postoperative pain: The case of inguinal herniorrhaphy. British Journal of Anaesthesia. 2005;**95**(1):69-76

[14] Massaron S, Bona S, Fumagalli U, Battafarano F, Elmore U, Rosati R. Analysis of post-surgical pain after inguinal hernia repair: A prospective study of 1,440 operations. Hernia. 2007;**11**(6):517-525

[15] Woo KP, Ellis RC, Maskal SM, Remulla D, Shukla P, Rosen AJ, et al. The association of permanent versus absorbable fixation on developing chronic post-herniorrhaphy groin pain in patients undergoing laparoscopic inguinal hernia repair. Surgical Endoscopy. 2024;**38**(6):3433-3440

[16] Olsson A, Sandblom G, Franneby U, Sondén A, Gunnarsson U, Dahlstrand U. Do postoperative complications correlate to chronic pain following inguinal hernia repair? A prospective cohort study from the Swedish Hernia Register. Hernia. 2023;**27**(1):21-29

[17] Reinpold WM, Nehls J, Eggert A. Nerve management and chronic pain

after open inguinal hernia repair: A prospective two phase study. Annals of Surgery. 2011;**254**(1):163-168

[18] Aasvang EK, Kehlet H. Persistent sensory dysfunction in pain-free herniotomy. Acta Anaesthesiologica Scandinavica. 2010;**54**(3):291-298

[19] Loos MJA, Roumen RMH, Scheltinga MRM. Classifying post-herniorrhaphy pain syndromes following elective inguinal hernia repair. World Journal of Surgery. 2007;**31**(9):1760-1765

[20] Hakeem A, Shanmugam V. Current trends in the diagnosis and management of post-herniorraphy chronic groin pain. World Journal of Gastrointestinal Surgery. 2011;**3**(6):73-81

[21] Heise CP, Starling JR. Mesh inguinodynia: A new clinical syndrome after inguinal herniorrhaphy? Journal of the American College of Surgeons. 1998;**187**(5):514-518

[22] Demirer S, Kepenekci I, Evirgen O, Birsen O, Tuzuner A, Karahuseyinoglu S, et al. The effect of polypropylene mesh on ilioinguinal nerve in open mesh repair of groin hernia. The Journal of Surgical Research. 2006;**131**(2):175-181

[23] Ducic I, West J, Maxted W. Management of chronic postoperative groin pain. Annals of Plastic Surgery. 2008;**60**(3):294-298

[24] Broin EO, Horner C, Mealy K, Kerin MJ, Gillen P, O'Brien M, et al. Meralgia paraesthetica following laparoscopic inguinal hernia repair. An anatomical analysis. Surgical Endoscopy. 1995;**9**(1):76-78

[25] Ducic I, Dellon AL. Testicular pain after inguinal hernia repair: An approach to resection of the genital branch of genitofemoral nerve. Journal of the American College of Surgeons. 2004;**198**(2):181-184

[26] Amid PK, Hiatt JR. New understanding of the causes and surgical treatment of postherniorrhaphy inguinodynia and orchalgia. Journal of the American College of Surgeons. 2007;**205**(2):381-385

[27] Tomašević-Todorović S. Central sensitization in patients with chronic musculoskeletal pain. Acta Clinica Croatica. 2023;**62**(Suppl. 4):102-106

[28] Latremoliere A, Woolf CJ. Central sensitization: A generator of pain hypersensitivity by central neural plasticity. The Journal of Pain. 2009;**10**(9):895-926

[29] Akui C, Kimura T, Hirose M. Associations between insomnia and central sensitization in cancer survivors undergoing opioid therapy for chronic cancer pain: A STROBE-compliant prospective cohort study. Medicine. 2022;**101**(38):e30845

[30] Ji R, Nackley A, Huh Y, Terrando N, Maixner W. Neuroinflammation and central sensitization in chronic and widespread pain. Anesthesiology. 2018;**129**(2):343-366

[31] Gottrup H, Andersen J, Arendt-Nielsen L, Jensen TS. Psychophysical examination in patients with post-mastectomy pain. Pain. 2000;**87**(3):275-284

[32] Liem MS, van Duyn EB, van der Graaf Y, van Vroonhoven TJ. Recurrences after conventional anterior and laparoscopic inguinal hernia repair: A randomized comparison. Annals of Surgery. 2003;**237**(1):136-141

[33] Eklund A, Montgomery A, Bergkvist L, Rudberg C. Chronic pain

5 years after randomized comparison of laparoscopic and lichtenstein inguinal hernia repair. British Journal of Surgery. 2010;**97**(4):600-608

[34] Nienhuijs SW, Boelens OB, Strobbe LJ. Pain after anterior mesh hernia repair. Journal of the American College of Surgeons. 2005;**200**(6):885-889

[35] Hoffmann H, Walther D, Bittner R, Köckerling F, Adolf D, Kirchhoff P. Smaller inguinal hernias are independent risk factors for developing chronic postoperative inguinal pain (CPIP): A registry-based multivariable analysis of 57, 999 patients. Annals of Surgery. 2020;**271**(4):756-764

[36] Huerta S, Timmerman C, Argo M, Favela J, Pham T, Kukreja S, et al. Open, laparoscopic, and robotic inguinal hernia repair: Outcomes and predictors of complications. The Journal of Surgical Research. 2019;**241**:119-127

[37] Fränneby U, Sandblom G, Nordin P, Nyrén O, Gunnarsson U. Risk factors for long-term pain after hernia surgery. Annals of Surgery. 2006;**244**(2):212-219

[38] Caumo W, Schmidt AP, Schneider CN, Bergmann J, Iwamoto CW, Adamatti LC, et al. Preoperative predictors of moderate to intense acute postoperative pain in patients undergoing abdominal surgery. Acta Anaesthesiologica Scandinavica. 2002;**46**(10):1265-1271

[39] Jakobsson E, Lundström KJ, Holmberg H, de la Croix H, Nordin P. Chronic pain after groin hernia surgery in women: A patient-reported outcome study based on data from the Swedish hernia register. Annals of Surgery. 2022;**275**(2):213-219

[40] Aasvang EK, Møhl B, Bay-Nielsen M, Kehlet H. Pain related sexual dysfunction after inguinal herniorrhaphy. Pain. 2006;**122**(3):258-263

[41] De la Fuente HA, Guadarrama-Sistos Vazquez S, Farhat S, Reddy NK, Trakhtenbroit MA, Echo A. The emerging role of MRI neurography in the diagnosis of chronic inguinal pain. Langenbeck's Archives of Surgery. 2023;**408**(1):319

[42] Alfieri S, Amid PK, Campanelli G, Izard G, Kehlet H, Wijsmuller AR, et al. International guidelines for prevention and management of post-operative chronic pain following inguinal hernia surgery. Hernia. 2011;**15**(3):239-249

[43] Bogduk N. Diagnostic nerve blocks in chronic pain. Best Practice & Research. Clinical Anaesthesiology. 2002;**16**(4):565-578

[44] Aasvang EK, Brandsborg B, Christensen B, Jensen TS, Kehlet H. Neurophysiological characterization of postherniotomy pain. Pain. 2008;**137**(1):173-181

[45] Amid PK. A 1-stage surgical treatment for postherniorrhaphy neuropathic pain: Triple neurectomy and proximal end implantation without mobilization of the cord. Archives of Surgery. 2002;**137**(1):100-104

[46] Amid PK. Causes, prevention, and surgical treatment of postherniorrhaphy neuropathic inguinodynia: Triple neurectomy with proximal end implantation. Hernia. 2004;**8**(4):343-349

[47] Madura JA, Madura JA 2nd, Copper CM, Worth RM. Inguinal neurectomy for inguinal nerve entrapment: An experience with 100 patients. American Journal of Surgery. 2005;**189**(3):283-287

[48] Miserez M, Peeters E, Aufenacker T, Bouillot JL, Campanelli G, Conze J,

et al. Update with level 1 studies of the European Hernia Society guidelines on the treatment of inguinal hernia in adult patients. Hernia. 2014;**18**(2):151-163

[49] Barazanchi AW, Fagan PV, Smith BB, Hill AG. Routine neurectomy of inguinal nerves during open onlay mesh hernia repair: A meta-analysis of randomized trials. Annals of Surgery. 2016;**264**(1):64-72

[50] Bakker WJ, Aufenacker TJ, Boschman JS, Burgmans JPJ. Lightweight mesh is recommended in open inguinal (Lichtenstein) hernia repair: A systematic review and meta-analysis. Surgery. 2020;**167**(3):581-589

[51] Öberg S, Andresen K, Klausen TW, Rosenberg J. Chronic pain after mesh versus nonmesh repair of inguinal hernias: A systematic review and a network meta-analysis of randomized controlled trials. Surgery. 2018;**163**(5):1151-1159

[52] Bullen NL, Hajibandeh S, Hajibandeh S, Smart NJ, Antoniou SA. Suture fixation versus self-gripping mesh for open inguinal hernia repair: A systematic review with meta-analysis and trial sequential analysis. Surgical Endoscopy. 2021;**35**(6):2480-2492

[53] Jeroukhimov I, Wiser I, Karasic E, Nesterenko V, Poluksht N, Lavy R, et al. Reduced postoperative chronic pain after tension-free inguinal hernia repair using absorbable sutures: A single-blind randomized clinical trial. Journal of the American College of Surgeons. 2014;**218**(1):102-107

[54] Tolver MA, Rosenberg J, Juul P, Bisgaard T. Randomized clinical trial of fibrin glue versus tacked fixation in laparoscopic groin hernia repair. Surgical Endoscopy. 2013;**27**(8):2727-2733

[55] Hoyuela C, Juvany M, Carvajal F, Veres A, Troyano D, Trias M, et al. Randomized clinical trial of mesh fixation with glue or sutures for Lichtenstein hernia repair. The British Journal of Surgery. 2017;**104**(6):688-694

Chapter 6

Post-Herniorrhaphy Pain

Hany Mohammed El-Hadi Shoukat Mohammed

Abstract

Although hernia repair is one of the oldest surgical procedures with accumulated experience over generations. However, post-herniorrhaphy pain remains a daily patient complaint at the surgical outpatient clinics. Post-herniorrhaphy pain is a type of chronic pain with a neuropathic element that can be disabling to many patients and interfering with their daily lives. Proper diagnosis of this condition is essential before choosing an appropriate management plan. Many treatment options are available including pharmacological, non-pharmacological, and interventional procedures. Pharmacological choices include simple analgesics, opioids, antidepressants, anti-epileptics, and steroids. Non-pharmacological approaches comprise psychotherapy, physiotherapy, acupuncture, and lifestyle modification. Interventional nerve blocks or surgical exploration with neurectomy can be employed for many cases.

Keywords: chronic inguinal pain, ilioinguinal nerve and iliohypogastric nerve, neuropathic pain, peripheral nerve blocks, neurectomy, inguinodynia, hernia

1. Introduction

Inguinal hernias represent the most common type of abdominal wall hernias, and consequently, inguinal hernia repair is the most performed surgical procedure worldwide. Today, lichtenstein tension-free open repair and endoscopic/laparoscopic repair are the surgical techniques that are mostly performed. Although post-operative complications after hernia surgery may be low, chronic post-operative pain carries a real challenge to patients, families, and physicians. Many factors can predispose inguinal hernia patients to post-operative pain chronicity. Young age, female gender, diabetic patients, smoking habits, improbably managed acute post-operative pain, poor surgical techniques, and mesh application are among the most common predisposing factors. Investigations should be carried out once post-herniorrhaphy syndrome is suspected to exclude recurrence as a cause of pain and to identify patients who need surgical management from non-surgical approaches. Inguinodynia is a type of chronic pain that should be managed by a multidisciplinary approach. Surgeons, pain physicians, physiotherapists, dietitians, interventional radiologists, and psychologists should be recruited to incorporate an ideal management plan. Unfortunately, there is no single management strategy or an agreed guideline. In many patients, selective or triple neurectomy may be the definitive cure.

2. Definition of post-herniorrhaphy pain

PHPS is a medical condition where pain persists after hernia surgery and may threaten the patient's quality of life. Post-herniorrhaphy pain is diagnosed when post-operative pain persists for more than 3 months and is not related to other causes [1, 2].

3. Incidence

Globally, more than 20 million patients are operated upon for hernia repair annually. Post-herniorrhaphy pain is one of the chronic post-surgical pains (CPSP). Up to 50% of patients report some degree of residual groin pain and discomfort at one year of post-operative follow-up. The incidence of moderate-to-severe post-herniorrhaphy pain is around 3–6% of the patients. However, some authors reported that the incidence of moderate-to-severe inguinodynia ranges from 10 to 12%. This variability in the reported frequencies may be attributed to the varying surgical techniques available to approach inguinal hernia repair and the inconsistent tools used to diagnose post-herniorrhaphy pain. Due to the relatively high incidence of chronic post-surgical pain, the risk of developing post-herniorrhaphy pain should be discussed preoperatively with the patients to obtain informed consent [1, 3, 4].

3.1 Inguinodynia in children and neonates

The rate of chronic post-operative pain after groin hernia repair is lower in children and adolescents compared with that in adults.

However, patients with repaired inguinal hernias in childhood may have chronic groin pain during their adulthood life [5, 6].

4. Nomenclature

Inguinodynia is a generic term used to describe chronic groin pain after hernia repair. Post-herniorrhaphy pain syndrome (PHPS) is a distinct expression employed by clinicians to label sustained pain suffering after hernia repair. It is also termed chronic post-operative inguinal pain (CPIP) and post-herniorrhaphy groin pain. Chronic inguinal neuralgia is another term used to describe this distressing condition [1, 2].

5. Nature of pain

This chronic pain lasts for more than 3 months after hernia repair. It is mainly a neuropathic type of pain. The proportion of PHPS patients who are diagnosed with a neuropathic origin of pain after hernia repair ranges from 28.7 to 64%. This wide discrepancy in the type of pain incidence may be related to the differences in the tools used to diagnose neuropathic pain in different studies.

Somatic (nociceptive) pain may originate from damage to the pubic tubercle or incorporation of the periosteum of the pubic tubercle during suturing or stapling of the mesh predisposing to chronic inflammation and pain [7, 8].

6. Etiology and pathogenesis

Post-herniorrhaphy inguinodynia is caused by a combination of neuropathic (direct nerve injury) and nociceptive (tissue injury and inflammation) etiological factors. Pathogenesis of pain can be linked to pain centralization, neuroplasticity, deafferentation hyperalgesia, and excitatory coupling between sympathetic and afferent nociceptive nerve fibers.

Many factors are postulated to explain the predisposition to the persistence of post-operative inguinal pain.

Injury to inguinal nerves with neuroma formation occurs after surgical manipulation, traction, incision, or thermal damage from cautery use. Mesh inflammatory reaction can lead to fibrotic changes and granuloma formation causing pain.

The most common causes of non-neuropathic etiologies of inguinodynia are mesh mass, exaggerated scar tissue, or recurrence of hernia.

Meshoma is the wadding or wrinkling of the mesh due to inadequate mesh fixation or the use of a large mesh that fails to stay flat. Meshoma may cause nerve entrapment or damage [1, 8–10]

7. Epidemiology and risk factors

Post-herniorrhaphy pain incidence is increased in young age, obesity, those who had preoperative pain, insufficiently treated post-operative pain, recurrent surgery, radiotherapy, chemotherapy, and patients with psychological disorders [1]. Common risk factors include the following:

1. Type of patients:

   The female gender appeared to have a greater chance of developing PHPS than the male patients. Older patients tend to commence chronic pain less frequently. Severe types of pain are more often experienced in younger patients below 50 years.

   Smoking and poor glycemic control are considered independent predictors of inguinodynia [3, 9].

2. Type of anesthesia:

   Local infiltration is advantageous over spinal and general anesthesia in having a lower incidence of post-herniorrhaphy pain. Ilioinguinal/iliohypogastric blockade is also advantageous to both general and spinal anesthesia for the prevention of inguinodynia [3, 9].

3. Existence of preoperative pain:

   Studies found that patients with a higher incidence of post-operative chronic pain are more likely to have preoperative pain, hence the importance of adequate perioperative pain management [3].

4. Acute post-operative pain and pre-emptive analgesia:

 Uncontrolled acute post-operative pain may predict the predisposition to chronic pain development. Post-operative complications such as hernia recurrence, infection, and hematoma may also play a role. Aggressive early pain management can reduce chronic pain prevalence [3, 9–11].

5. Surgical techniques:

 Ilioinguinal nerve injury during surgery is an important factor influencing chronic pain. Debate continues to occur in the literature concerning the utility of elective transection of the nerve. Some authors believe that nerve preservation would minimize chronic pain incidence. At the same time, others suggested that elective intraoperative ligation of the ilioinguinal nerve will be associated with a little risk. It is recommended that all three inguinal nerves should be identified intraoperatively and preserved to prevent chronic pain. Failure to do so could lead to accidental nerve injury, entrapment, or suturing initiating severe pain post-operatively.

 The site at which the nerve divided could influence the generation of pain. Distal resection of the nerve leaves most of the nerve exposed with the possibility of neuroma formation. Division of the nerve if to be performed should be proximal to the site where it exits from the retroperitoneum.

 However, some advocate identifying the five nerves involved in groin innervation and preserving them during herniorrhaphy operation. These five nerves include the ilioinguinal nerve, the iliohypogastric nerve, the genitofemoral nerve, the lateral cutaneous nerve of the thigh, and the femoral nerve. The common nerve trapped in the scar tissue formed between the mesh and underlying muscles is the iliohypogastric nerve.

 During the minimally invasive techniques, the lateral cutaneous nerve of the thigh, the femoral branch of the genitofemoral nerve, and the femoral nerve are at greater risk of accidental injury. "Triangle of pain" is a theoretical region identified during laparoscopy and bounded by the gonadal vessels, iliopubic tract, and the peritoneum. Identifying this triangle during laparoscopic inguinal hernia repair is essential to avoid injuries to nerves that pass through that triangle.

 Suters and staples carry a greater risk of developing post-operative pain than other mesh-fixing materials. Fibrin glue is used for atraumatic mesh fixation. The incidence of chronic groin pain, foreign body sensation, and groin numbness is reduced when fibrin glue is used instead of sutures [3, 8, 10–12].

6. Laparoscopic surgery versus open surgery:

 Laparoscopic hernia repair is generally associated with less post-operative pain than open repairs. This advantage may be related to less dissection and tissue trauma to the ilioinguinal and iliohypogastric nerves. Inconsistent reports show a higher incidence of inguinodynia following open hernia repair, particularly with an anterior approach, compared with laparoscopic or robotic hernia repair through the posterior approach.

There are two main approaches for laparoscopic herniorrhaphy: the total extra-peritoneal (TEP) and preperitoneal transabdominal (TAPP) approaches. TEP and TAPP are techniques used also in bilateral inguinal hernias repair. Applying mesh without fixation in these cases appeared to lower the incidence of chronic post-operative pain.

Laparoscopic herniorrhaphy with the use of a tacker can cause nerve entrapment due to misplaced tacks.

Minimally invasive techniques using robotic-assisted surgery carry the same incidence of chronic pain [3, 8, 10, 13].

7. Mesh type, size, and weight:

Polypropylene meshes are commonly used for tension-free repair. Polypropylene as a synthetic material induces granulomatous reactions that encapsulate the mesh. Experimental research demonstrated that when a polypropylene mesh contacts peripheral nerve tissue; myelin degeneration, edema, fibrosis, and neuroma formation can precipitate neuralgia. However, these findings lack strong evidence.

Light macroporous (pores>75 micrometers) polypropylene meshes are preferred over heavy microporous (pores <10 micrometers) materials as the former creates a sufficient inflammatory response, tissue incorporation, and lesser incidence of foreign body sensation. Although the light biocompatible meshes were designed to reduce the foreign body reaction, they carried the same potential for post-operative chronic groin pain as traditional meshes.

The method by which the mesh is fixed has been found to impact the incidence of CPSP. The use of cyanoacrylate glue (Histoacryl) or a self-gripping mesh (Progrip) did not appear to reduce the risk of post-operative pain and chronic pain [3, 8, 10].

8. Recurrent cases:

Surgery for recurrent hernias may carry a greater surgical difficulty. Thus, the potential for persistence or even deterioration of pain is increased with the second surgery [10].

9. Psychologic predisposition:

Patients with a preoperative psychologic vulnerability are at increased risk of post-operative inguinodynia. The resultant lower pain threshold in these emotionally unstable patients could explain this [8].

10. Genetic predisposition:

People differ in their susceptibility to the experience of pain, as well as their response to analgesics due to inherited factors. This difference in genetic predisposition makes patients different in their sensitivity to nociceptive pain [10].

8. Clinical picture and presentation

8.1 Criteria of pain

Pain is not necessary to begin during the early post-operative days, but some patients may present with late-onset pain after a relatively long period of being symptom-free.

Patients may complain of any feature of neuropathic pain. Hyperalgesia, hypoesthesia, dysesthesia, or allodynia may be elicited at the surgical incision site or territory.

When the genitofemoral nerve is affected, testicular pain or labial pain arises.

Neuropathic pain presentation varies from a dull aching to sharp shooting pain traveling along the distribution of inguinal nerves. Pain can be elicited by wound site touching, tapping the area of tenderness, or tapping the medial aspect of the antero-superior iliac spine. Also, pain can be triggered by walking, exercise, deep breathing, coughing, bowel activity, hip hyperextension, or twisting. Conversely, pain is usually relieved by bed rest or flexion of the thigh.

Groin pain can radiate to the upper leg, scrotum, or back. Some male patients may complain of testicular or ejaculatory pain, while female may complain of labial pain. Trigger points can be found in the vicinity of the scar tissue. Also, some may report numbness over the thigh or groin.

Inflammatory pain usually presents with throbbing quality and heat hyperalgesia and tends to subside over an expected period. Inflammatory pain is not accompanied by sensory or motor deficits.

Nociceptive (somatic) pain is usually dull aching continuous type of pain, of little intensity, and may be diffuse, localized, or projected to surrounding regions. Nociceptive pain develops acutely and tends to diminish over time, while neuropathic pain continues to persist for longer times.

Distinguishing neuropathic from the nociceptive origin of pain may be impractical as symptoms of both usually overlap making clinical differentiation difficult [1, 3, 8, 10, 12].

8.2 Location of pain

Commonly patients reported pain in the groin, scar, or both. However, others may report pain at unexpected locations, such as the lower abdomen, genitalia, and thigh. These unexpected sites have no apparent relation to the innervation of the surgical field. The development of pain in unforeseen locations, while pain is absent in expected ones, can be explained by the inflammatory processes following surgery and not merely the nerve damage [7, 10].

8.3 Pain intensity

Chronic groin pain following inguinal herniorrhaphy ranges from mild to severe form of pain that can be debilitating [8, 10].

8.4 Impairment of everyday activities

This chronic pain can cause functional limitations in daily tasks such as sitting, standing up, performing sports, going up and down stairs, and driving a car. PHPS impairs the patient's work capabilities, and social life, and causes sleep disturbances.

DOI: http://dx.doi.org/10.5772/intechopen.1006681

Moreover, chronic groin pain contributes to erectile dysfunction and ejaculatory pain. Around one-third of men with inguinodynia had sexual dysfunction [1, 3, 10, 12].

9. Evaluation of and diagnosis of post-herniorrhaphy pain

9.1 History

Patients should be interviewed and asked about the onset and quality of pain, radiation of pain, what makes symptoms improve, and what causes symptoms to worsen. Surgical history includes the type of hernia (i.e., direct versus indirect), type of surgery (i.e., open versus laparoscopic), and history of post-operative complications [10].

9.2 Physical examinations

The first step in managing chronic pain following inguinal hernia repair starts with a formal and proper patient examination. General and surgical examination should include evaluation of the inguinal region. Clinical tests aim to diagnose the type of nerve (**Table 1**) entrapped, for example, in case of ilioinguinal nerve entrapment; hyperextension and twisting the trunk away from the affected side will elicit symptoms. Moreover, urological and gynecologic evaluation must follow to exclude underlying testicular and gynecological pathologies [10].

Nerve	Innervation	Location
Ilioinguinal nerve (T12, T1)	Sensory to: • Proximal & medial thigh • Mons pubis & labia majora • Root of penis & upper scrotum	Go along the spermatic cord
Ibiohypogastric nerve (T12, L1):		
• Anterior cutaneous branch	Sensory to hypogastric region	Passes between the sponeurosis & internal oblique; to accompany the spermatic cord
• Lateral cutaneous branch	Sensory to gluteal region	Pierces the internal & external oblique above the iliac crest
Genitofemoral nerve (L1, L2):		
• Genital branch	Sensory to mons & scrotum/ labia	Joins the spermatic cord through the internal ring
• Femoral branch	Sensory to the anterolateral thigh	Passes with the external iliac artery
Lateral femoral cutaneous nerve (L2, L3)	Sensory to the anterolateral thigh	Passes under the inguinal ligament
Femoral nerve (L2, L3)	Motor innervation to quadriceps femoris	Passes under the inguinal ligament
	Sensory to the anterior thigh	

Table 1.
Sensory and motor impairment in inguinal neuropathies [10].

9.2.1 Pain assessment tools

Neuropathic pain can be evaluated by using questionnaires, quantitative sensory testing (QST), and dermatosensory mapping [7, 14].

a. *EuraHS Quality of Life (QoL):*

The EuraHS-QoL score (**Figure 1**) is a hernia-specific quality-of-life assessment tool developed and validated by the European Hernia Society. The EuraHS-QoL Scale has nine questions, with a total score ranging from 0 to 90. The patient is scored on an 11-point scale from 0 to 10. A score of 0 means the patient is in the best condition while 10 for the worst condition. The EuraHS-QoL score questions have three domains: pain (0–30), restriction of activities (0–40), and esthetical discomfort (0–20) [15].

b. *DN-4, for neuropathic pain diagnosis*:

DN4 (Douleur Neuropathique en 4 Questions) is a screening tool designed to assess neuropathic pain. DN-4 consists of an interview questionnaire (DN4-interview) and bedside physical tests. The DN-4 questionnaire (DN4-interview) consists of four groups of questions: First group assesses the characteristics of pain (burning, painful cold, electric shocks), and second group evaluates

EuraHS-QoL Preoperative

Pain at the site of hernia [0 = no pain, 10 = worst pain imaginable]												
While lying down at rest	0	1	2	3	4	5	6	7	8	9	10	
During activities (walking, biking, sports)	0	1	2	3	4	5	6	7	8	9	10	
Worst pain felt during the last week	0	1	2	3	4	5	6	7	8	9	10	
Restrictions of daily activities because of pain or discomfort at the site of the hernia [0 = no pain, 10 = worst pain imaginable, x = if you do not perform the activity]												
Inside the house	0	1	2	3	4	5	6	7	8	9	10	x
Outside the house (walking, biking, driving)	0	1	2	3	4	5	6	7	8	9	10	x
During sports	0	1	2	3	4	5	6	7	8	9	10	x
During heavy labour	0	1	2	3	4	5	6	7	8	9	10	x
Cosmetic discomfort [0 = very beautiful, 10 = extremely ugly]												
The shape of the abdomen	0	1	2	3	4	5	6	7	8	9	10	
The site of the hernia	0	1	2	3	4	5	6	7	8	9	10	

EuraHS-QoL Postoperative

Pain at the site of hernia repair [0 = no pain, 10 = worst pain imaginable]												
While lying down at rest	0	1	2	3	4	5	6	7	8	9	10	
During activities (walking, biking, sports)	0	1	2	3	4	5	6	7	8	9	10	
Worst pain felt during the last week	0	1	2	3	4	5	6	7	8	9	10	
Restrictions of daily activities because of pain or discomfort at the site of the hernia repair [0 = no pain, 10 = worst pain imaginable, x = if you do not perform the activity]												
Inside the house	0	1	2	3	4	5	6	7	8	9	10	x
Outside the house (walking, biking, driving)	0	1	2	3	4	5	6	7	8	9	10	x
During sports	0	1	2	3	4	5	6	7	8	9	10	x
During heavy labour	0	1	2	3	4	5	6	7	8	9	10	x
Cosmetic discomfort [0 = very beautiful, 10 = extremely ugly]												
The shape of the abdomen	0	1	2	3	4	5	6	7	8	9	10	
The site of the hernia & the scars	0	1	2	3	4	5	6	7	8	9	10	

Figure 1.
The EuraHS-QoL score [15].

other symptoms associated with pain (tingling, pins and needles, numbness, itching). Three bedside neurological examinations are done in the painful area (touch hypoesthesia using a soft brush or cotton swab, pinprick hypoesthesia using disposable examination pins such as Von Frey filaments, and tactile dynamic allodynia using a soft brush). For scoring, the 10 items DN-4 tool, 0 is given to each negative item, while 1 is given to each positive item (total score range 0–10).
For neuropathic pain to be diagnosed, the patient should earn a total score of 4 with at least a score of 3 on the DN4-interview questionnaire [1].

c. *The Brief Pain Inventory (BPI) for severity, analgesic use, and interference with activities:*

The Brief Pain Inventory (BPI) is a quick and easy means of measuring pain intensity and its effects on patients' lives (**Figure 2**). It is primarily developed for the assessment of cancer-related pain; however, it can be applied to many types of chronic pain.

BPI covers five fields of functioning. The patient is asked to rate the intensity of pain using a numeric scale of 0 to 10 and report it as being worst, least, and average. A score of 0 means "no pain," while a score of 10 means "pain as bad as you can imagine." Then, the patient is requested to document the interference of pain on seven quality-of-life domains including general activity, walking, mood, sleep, work, relations with other persons, and enjoyment of life.

Each point of the seven domains will be answered as "does not interfere" or "interferes completely." The BPI is available in short and long forms [12, 16].

d. *The SF-12 questionnaire for QoL:*

Short Form 12-item survey (SF-12) is an instrument used for evaluation of health-related quality of life (HRQL). It consists of a 12-item questionnaire grouped into two main domains: the physical component summary (PCS-12) scores and the mental component summary (MCS-12) scores. The PCS-12 domain involves physical functioning (PF), role-physical (RP), bodily pain (BP), and general health (GH) subdomains, while the MCS-12 domain involves vitality (VT), social functioning (SF), role-emotional (RE), and mental health (MH) subdomains. Each item's raw scores range from 1 to 6 with a total score transformed into a 0–100 scale. A higher score indicates a good health status [17].

e. *Visual analogue scale (VAS):*

This simple pain assessment tool uses a scale of 10 cm in length, where 0 means no pain and 10 means severe pain [16].

9.2.2 Pain maps

Surgeons use dermatome inguinal mapping tests to map the pain distribution on patients' skin. Pain mapping can identify areas with hypothesis, numbness, and

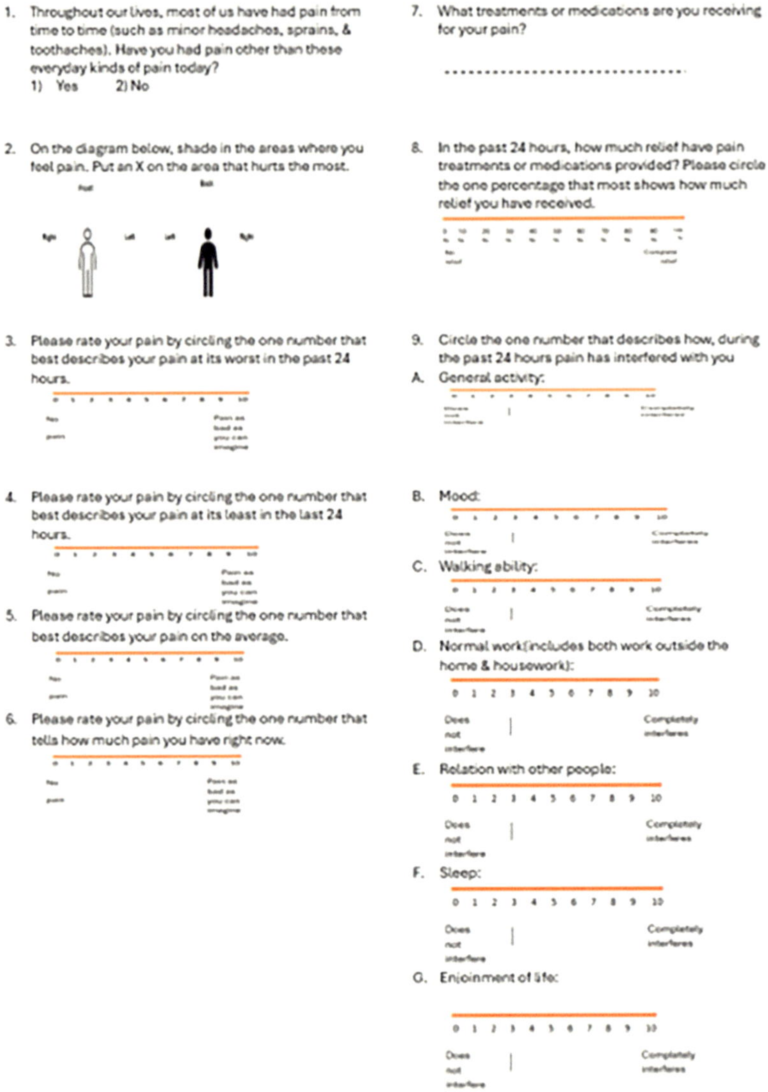
1. Throughout our lives, most of us have had pain from time to time (such as minor headaches, sprains, & toothaches). Have you had pain other than these everyday kinds of pain today?
1) Yes 2) No

2. On the diagram below, shade in the areas where you feel pain. Put an X on the area that hurts the most.

3. Please rate your pain by circling the one number that best describes your pain at its worst in the past 24 hours.

4. Please rate your pain by circling the one number that best describes your pain at its least in the last 24 hours.

5. Please rate your pain by circling the one number that best describes your pain on the average.

6. Please rate your pain by circling the one number that tells how much pain you have right now.

7. What treatments or medications are you receiving for your pain?

....

8. In the past 24 hours, how much relief have pain treatments or medications provided? Please circle the one percentage that most shows how much relief you have received.

9. Circle the one number that describes how, during the past 24 hours pain has interfered with you

A. General activity:

B. Mood:

C. Walking ability:

D. Normal work(includes both work outside the home & housework):

0 1 2 3 4 5 6 7 8 9 10

Does not interfere | Completely interferes

E. Relation with other people:

0 1 2 3 4 5 6 7 8 9 10

Does not interfere | Completely interferes

F. Sleep:

0 1 2 3 4 5 6 7 8 9 10

Does not interfere | Completely interferes

G. Enjoinment of life:

0 1 2 3 4 5 6 7 8 9 10

Does not interfere | Completely interferes

Figure 2.
The Brief Pain Inventory (BPI) [16].

pain sensation (**Figures 3** and **4**). Exposure and examination of the groin, abdomen, thigh, and genitals are made, and then, a mark is applied by a surgical marker over the examined skin. A "zero" sign can be used to indicate areas with no pain, and a "minus" sign is used to indicate a numb area, while a "plus or x" sign is used to mark the area with pain. By generating pain maps identification of the involved nerves can be easily outlined. Photos can be taken of these maps and comparisons can be made between pain location and intensity before and after initiation of treatment [14].

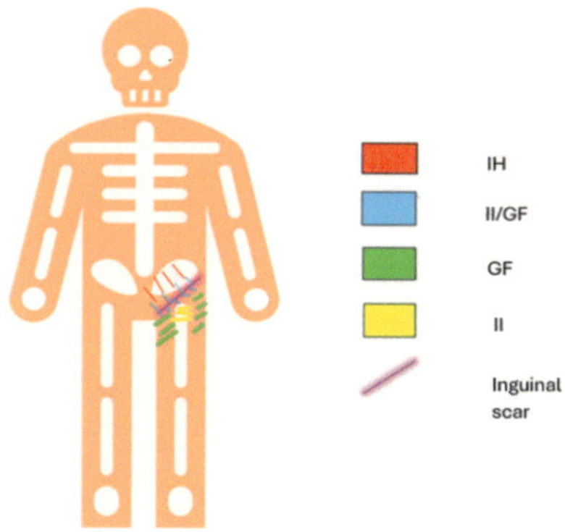

Figure 3.
Dermatomes mapping test. IH = iliohypogastric, II = ilioinguinal, and GF = genitofemoral nerves [14].

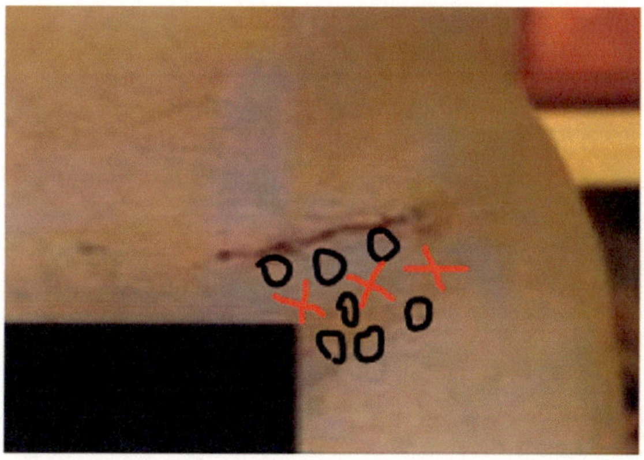

Figure 4.
Dermatomal distribution of inguinal nerves. O = hypoesthesia or numbness. X = pain [14].

9.3 Investigations

Ultrasound and CT examination can diagnose occult recurrences and non-neuropathic sources of pain. MRI can recognize abnormal mesh position and the presence of recurrence. MR neurography can identify the accurate site of injured nerves. Both US and MRI can confirm the presence of neuroma. Imaging studies can diagnose osteitis pubis as a preventable cause of pain induced by a suture or staples placed into the pubic tubercle [10].

9.4 Diagnostic algorithm

Any patient having persistent groin pain for more than 6–8 weeks following inguinal hernia repair despite standard pain management should be suspected to have post-herniorrhaphy neuralgia.

9.4.1 Confirm the diagnosis

Clinical examination will confirm the diagnosis if the following three criteria are positive:

1. History of burning or stabbing pain near the groin incision radiating along a specific inguinal nerve distribution.

2. Sensory impairment along the distribution of a specific groin nerve.

3. Peripheral nerve block alleviates the pain.

Groin nerve blocks are used for diagnostic and curative purposes. Injection of long-acting local anesthetic with steroids is commonly performed. However, a negative diagnostic peripheral nerve block does not exclude the diagnosis, as the spread of local anesthetic may be impaired in the presence of mesh fibrosis.

9.4.2 Recognition of the possible etiology and identification of the involved nerve

Imaging studies may help confirm the diagnosis, exclude recurrence and other pain causes, identify nerve abnormalities, and differentiate between patients requiring surgical and non-surgical management.

Algorithms have been developed for diagnosis and treatment (**Figures** 5 and **6**) [10].

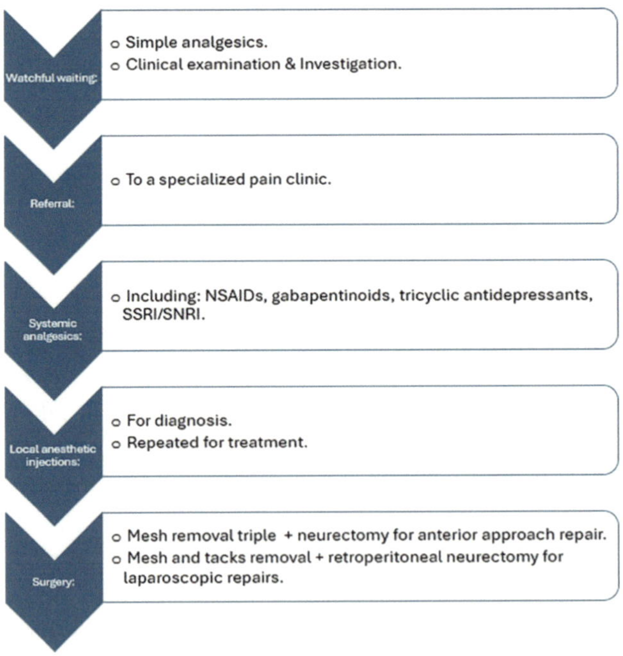

Figure 5.
A scaled approach for treatment options for chronic pain following inguinal hernia repair. *NSAID: nonsteroidal anti-inflammatory drug; SSRI, selective serotonin reuptake inhibitor; SNRI, serotonin-norepinephrine reuptake inhibitor [18].*

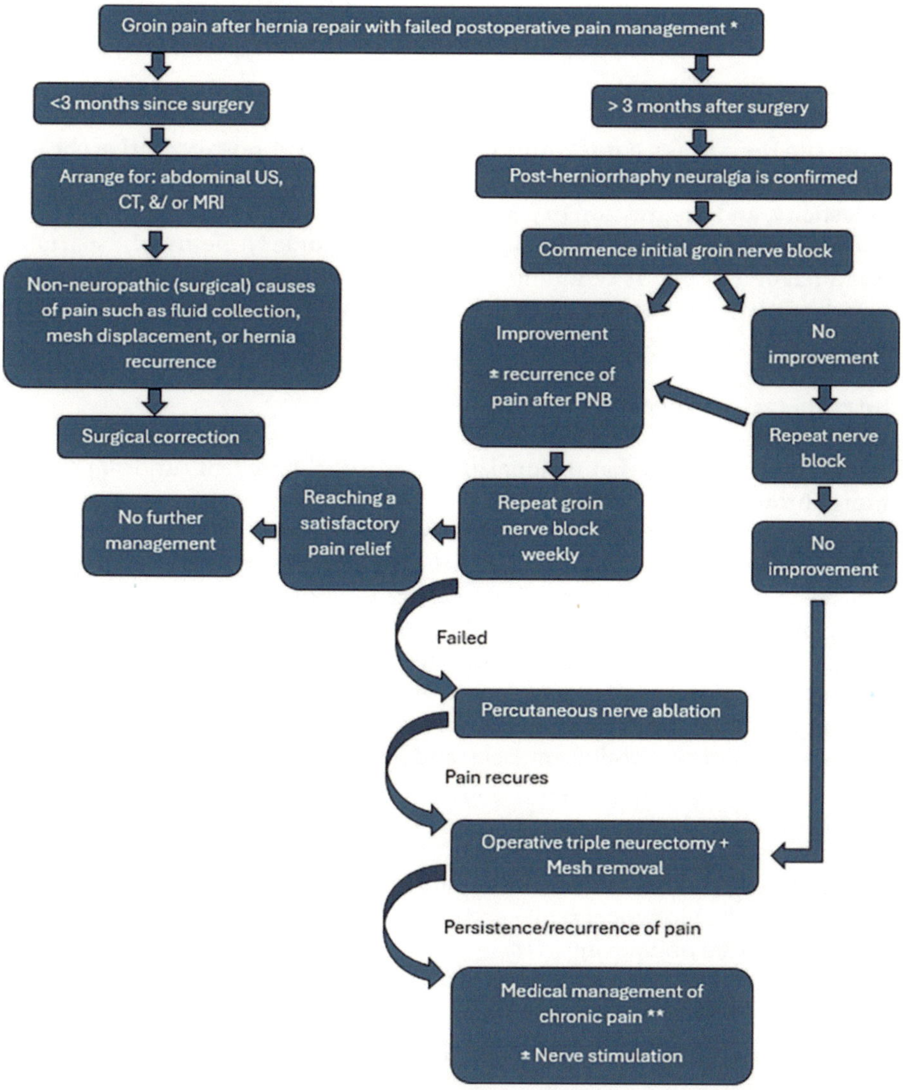

Figure 6.
Management algorithm for post-herniorrhaphy groin pain. *US: ultrasound; CT: computed tomography; MRI: magnetic resonance imaging; NSAIDs: nonsteroidal anti-inflammatory drugs. *Post-operative pain management includes NSAIDs and/or narcotic medications, as well as nonpharmacologic measures such as rest and icing of the groin area. ** Chronic pain management includes anti-epileptics (e.g., gabapentin or progabalin) or antidepressants (e.g., duloxetine) [10].*

9.5 Differential diagnosis

The pain of post-herniorrhaphy neuralgia should be differentiated from the following:

- Other causes of groin pain such as hernia recurrence, mesh infection or displacement, hematoma, fluid collection, and osteitis pubis.

- Other causes of lower abdominal pain such as diseases of the spine, lumbosacral plexus, and peripheral nerves of the lower abdomen [10].

10. Prevention

10.1 Preoperative management

Acute pain therapy is a cornerstone in the prevention of post-operative chronic pain. Adequate control of post-operative pain may prevent central sensitization, neuroplasticity, and progression to post-operative pain.

Perioperative multimodal analgesia approaches include N-methyl-d-aspartate receptor antagonists such as ketamine, COX inhibitors, gabapentin or pregabalin, corticosteroids, and regional blocks. Diclofenac prescription as a type of NSAID in the 1st week after surgery was shown to prevent the development of inguinodynia [3, 11].

10.2 Intraoperative preventive strategy

Several studies showed that regional anesthesia could prevent surgical pain from becoming chronic.

Comprehensive knowledge of the inguinal region anatomy with cautious surgical techniques preserving the inguinal nerves is the basis for the prevention of inguinodynia. Some recommend performing inguinal ultrasound to identify the relevant nerves.

During open herniorrhaphy, the following maneuvers and surgical techniques are recommended intraoperatively to minimize nerve injury: avoid unnecessary subcutaneous tissue dissection, avoid cremasteric muscle destruction, identify and preserve all the inguinal nerves, particularly the ilioinguinal nerve, avoid sutures in the lower edge of the internal oblique muscle, and avoid tightening of the inguinal ring. Avoiding nerve damage by laparoscopic approach may help to decrease post-operative chronic pain development.

Intraoperatively, the surgeon can identify the ilioinguinal nerve lateral to the internal ring, the genital branch of the genitofemoral in the lateral crus of the internal ring. In contrast, the iliohypogastric nerve can be identified in the plane between the external and internal oblique muscles.

Selection of a light (≤ 50 g/m^2) mesh, the use of fibrin glue rather than suture or tack, and the use of absorbable sutures to secure a mesh when glue is not available all can reduce the incidence of post-operative pain [3, 8–10].

10.2.1 Prophylactic neurectomy

Identification and preservation of all inguinal nerves passing through the operative field during open hernia repair has been advocated as a standard practice. However, some surgeons support prophylactic ilioinguinal neurectomy to reduce the incidence of post-operative chronic inguinal pain. Nevertheless, studies failed to find a statistical significance in the incidence of inguinodynia. Prophylactic neurectomy may result in loss of inguinal sensation and groin numbness.

Thus, the decision for groin nerve preservation versus scarification should be made on individual basis with a clear explanation of potential outcomes [3, 8–10].

11. Management

Due to the multifactorial etiology of the disease, there are no globally accepted guidelines or consensus for the management of ingunodynia. Careful diagnosis and exclusion of other causes of pain especially hernia recurrence is an essential step before starting the treatment plan [10].

11.1 Conservative management

The first line of treatment comprises a watchful waiting strategy with or without analgesia. Pain usually improves in many cases.

Modalities include oral analgesics, gabapentinoids, pregabalin, tricyclic antidepressants, selective serotonin reuptake inhibitor, serotonin/norepinephrine reuptake inhibitors, regional nerve blocks, and acupuncture. Local applications of lidocaine or capsaicin patches have been tried in some cases but failed to find a significant benefit.

Selective nerve blocks can be done for both diagnostic and therapeutic purposes. Some patients may benefit from combined injections of lidocaine, corticosteroids, and hyaluronic acid.

Cognitive behavioral therapy can be used alone or in combination with nerve block techniques. Spinal cord stimulation by using an implanted device has been tried in some cases.

Lifestyle modifications including healthy diet, exercise, and smoking cessation are proven to improve the condition [3, 8–10].

11.2 Neurectomy

If the response to a specific groin nerve block was transient and the pain recurred, this will indicate the need for a nerve sacrifice procedure. Nerve sacrifice can be achieved by either percutaneous nerve ablation or surgical neurectomy [10].

11.2.1 Nerve ablation procedure

Nerve ablation is considered a minimally invasive procedure with minimal side effects less than neurectomy. Nerve ablation should be tried as a first line for managing patients with refractory responses to repeated nerve blocks. The technique of nerve ablation is like that of nerve block but with an injection of either phenol or alcohol to destroy the offending nerve ending permanently. Percutaneous nerve ablation may fail to relieve permanent pain as nerve regeneration may occur in many cases.

Cryoablation and radiofrequency ablation are alternative techniques of percutaneous nerve ablation. Pulsed radiofrequency gained popularity as a technique for nerve destruction. It can be applied at either the level of peripheral nerves or at the dorsal root ganglia [7, 10].

11.2.2 Surgical management

Surgical management appeared to be the most effective treatment option for persistent groin pain in patients with post-herniorrhaphy neuralgia. There is no evidence-based nor optimal strategy for surgical treatment of chronic pain following inguinal hernia repair.

Surgical options include laparoscopic mesh removal with or without retroperitoneal neurectomies.

11.2.2.1 Indication

Surgical intervention is indicated when non-surgical measures including nerve block/ablation fail to control the pain. A surgical treatment plan will be based on the character of the pain, the original repair technique, confirmation of recurrence, the presence of meshoma, and the method and type of fixation material.

Surgical management includes exploration with mesh excision, neuroma identification and excision, and surgical neurectomy.

11.2.2.2 Neurolysis

Freeing the nerve by surgical neurolysis only has been associated with a high failure rate.

11.2.2.3 Surgical neurectomy

Neurectomy can be either selective or triple neurectomy. It can also be performed laparoscopically or by an open technique. Some authors recommend an open approach when the original triggering surgery was open surgery, while a laparoscopic approach is recommended when the original surgery was laparoscopic.

11.2.2.3.1 Triple neurectomy

Groin exploration with triple neurectomy that involves the ilioinguinal, iliohypogastric, and genitofemoral results in permanent pain relief in about 90% of patients. However, the genital branch of the genitofemoral nerve must be preserved in females to preserve the sensory supply to labia majora. Although triple neurectomy is safe and recommended by many,it is an aggressive procedure with an increased risk of a larger area of anesthesia. A complete loss of sensation over the distributions of the resected nerves is a common morbidity of triple neurectomy. Thus, selective neurectomy is preferred by some surgeons over triple neurectomy.

The surgical neurectomy procedure involves nerve identification, dissection, and resection of the entire length of a nerve. The remaining smooth ends of the nerve should be ligated, cauterized, or implanted within a healthy muscle or retroperitoneal tissue. In the case of orchialgia, paravasal nerve resection may also be needed.

Patients undergoing laparoscopic triple neurectomy procedures should be informed about the possible post-operative complications. These complications may include abdominal wall laxity from the oblique muscle denervation, persistent numbness, female labia numbness, loss of a male cremasteric reflex, interference with normal sexual sensation, testicular atrophy, and failure to identify the inguinal nerves.

- Open triple neurectomy technique:

  Triple neurectomy by an open approach has many challenges and difficulties such as difficult access through the scarred tissues, intractable identification of the three inguinal nerves at the reoperated inguinal canal tissues, and the potential to disrupt the previous repair or injure the spermatic cord.

- Endoscopic/laparoscopic triple neurectomy technique:

Endoscopic triple neurectomy can be approached through a transabdominal or extraperitoneal (retroperitoneal) approach. Laparoscopic retroperitoneal triple neurectomies are the preferred definitive treatment of chronic inguinal neuralgia in the absence of both recurrence and meshoma. Laparoscopic retroperitoneal triple neurectomy is a minimally invasive technique that allows proximal division of main trunks of the IIN, IHN, and GFN at the lumbar plexus origin.

After anesthesia induction, the patient is placed on lateral decubitus with the involved side being the uppermost one. The plane between the iliac crest and lower costal margin is exposed by flexion of the operating table. At 4 cm proximal to the iliac crest in the midaxillary line, a transverse incision is done. Then, dissection through external oblique muscle and abdominal wall muscles is made to reach the retroperitoneal space. Thereafter, a 12-mm trochar is inserted at that plane and through the incision CO2 insufflation starts. To identify the nerves, the quadratus lumborum and psoas muscle should be identified first.

Resection of the common trunk of the ilioinguinal and iliohypogastric nerves can be achieved between the quadratus lumborum and psoas muscles. These nerves should be resected as distal as possible. The genitofemoral nerve can be identified as penetrating the middle part of psoas muscle, while the lateral cutaneous femoral nerve can be seen lateral to the psoas muscle. After neurectomies, the mesh can be removed through a transabdominal approach after turning the patient to the supine position [3, 7–10, 19, 20].

11.2.2.3.2 Selective neurectomy

Although selective neurectomy avoids the permanent sensory deficit caused by triple neurectomy, it may be less effective in relieving chronic pain than a triple neurectomy.

- Mesh removal

Removal of the mesh is sufficient to reverse the chronic pain in many cases but accidental nerve damage during the procedure leads to post-operative pain persistence. So, it is recommended to combine neurectomy with mesh removal. Mesh removal alone but without neurectomy does not lead to life-long pain relief. Surgical treatment typically includes mesh removal and replacement with a new one. Mesh removal without replacement can predispose patients to develop a recurrent hernia. Some authors advocate the placement of the new mesh in an opposite location to the old one, for example, in the preperitoneal space. If the original repair was open, the new mesh is recommended to be inserted laparoscopically and if the previous repair was laparoscopic, the following repair is advised to be open.

Laparoscopically repaired hernia causing chronic pain due to improperly placed tacks requires laparoscopic re-exploration and removing the offending tacks [3, 8–10, 19, 20].

Author details

Hany Mohammed El-Hadi Shoukat Mohammed
Department of Anesthesia, Surgical ICU and Pain Management, Cairo University, Cairo, Egypt

*Address all correspondence to: oblfollower_2001@yahoo.com

References

[1] Ergönenç T, Beyaz SG, Özocak H, Palabıyık O, Altıntoprak F. Persistent postherniorrhaphy pain following inguinal hernia repair: A cross-sectional study of prevalence, pain characteristics, and effects on quality of life. International Journal of Surgery. 2017;**46**:126-132. DOI: 10.1016/j.ijsu.2017.08.588

[2] Krpata DM. Management of chronic postoperative inguinal pain. Review article. Surgical Clinics of North America. 2023;**103**(5):889-900. DOI: 10.1016/j.suc.2023.04.003

[3] Barbosa CDA, Oliveira DC, De-Melo-Delgado NM, Mafra JGDA, Santos RSD, Moreira WC. Inguinodynia: Review of predisposing factors and management. Revista do Colégio Brasileiro de Cirurgiões. 2021;**47**(e20202607):47. Available from: https://www.scielo.br/j/rcbc/a/HTDSwFqXbmntY9dc8fSvJVb/?lang=pt. DOI: 10.1590/0100-6991e-20202607

[4] Sivarajah V, Farquharson B, Mahdi S, Cathcart P, Jeyarajah S. Chronic groin pain following open inguinal hernia repair: Has consenting practice improved? Annals of the Royal College of Surgeons of England. 2021;**103**(1):5-9. Available from: https://pubmed.ncbi.nlm.nih.gov/32981334/https://doi.org/10.1308/rcsann.2020.0184

[5] Reistrup H, Andresen K, Rosenberg J. Low incidence of recurrence and chronic pain after groin hernia repair in adolescents: A systematic review and meta-analysis. Langenbeck's Archives of Surgery. 26 May 2023;**408**(1):211. DOI: 10.1007/s00423-023-02947-9

[6] Zendejas B, Zarroug AE, Erben YM, Holley CT, Harmsen WS, Huebner M, et al. Impact of childhood inguinal hernia repair in adulthood: A fifty year follow-up. Journal of the American College of Surgeons. 2010;**211**(3):S71-S71. DOI: 10.1016/j.jamcollsurg.2010.06.184

[7] Bande D, Moltó L, Pereira JA, Montes A. Chronic pain after groin hernia repair: Pain characteristics and impact on quality of life. BMC Surgery. Jul 2020;**20**(1):147. DOI: 10.1186/s12893-020-00805-9

[8] Ferzli G, Edwards ED, Al-Khoury GE, Hardin RE. Postherniorrhaphy groin pain and how to avoid it. Surgical Clinics of North America. 2008;**88**(1):203-216. DOI: 10.1016/j.suc.2007.10.006

[9] Chen DC, Hiatt JR, Amid PK. Operative management of refractory neuropathic inguinodynia by a laparoscopic retroperitoneal approach. JAMA Surgery. 2013;**148**(10):962-967. DOI: 10.1001/jamasurg.2013.3189

[10] Bonwich JB, Rosen M, Chen W. Post-Herniorrhaphy Groin Pain. Wellesley, Massachusetts: UpToDate; 2024. Available from: info@uptodate.com; www.uptodate.com

[11] Manangi M, Shivashankar S, Vijayakumar A. Chronic pain after inguinal hernia repair. International Scholarly Research Notices. 2014;**2014**:1-6. DOI: 10.1155/2014/839681

[12] Hakeem A. Inguinodynia following lichtenstein tension-free hernia repair: A review. World Journal of Gastroenterology. 2011;**17**(14):1791. Available from: https://www.ncbi.nlm.nih.gov/pmc/articles/PMC3080712/. DOI: 10.3748/wjg.v17.i14.1791

[13] Rodrigues-Gonçalves V, Verdaguer-Tremolosa M, Martínez-López P, et al. Open vs. robot-assisted preperitoneal inguinal hernia repair. Are they truly clinically different? Hernia. 2024;**28**:1355-1363. DOI: 10.1007/s10029-024-03050-8

[14] Cirocchi R, Mercurio I, Nazzaro C, De Sol A, Boselli C, Rettagliata G, et al. Dermatome mapping test in the analysis of anatomo-clinical correlations after inguinal hernia repair. BMC Surgery. 7 Dec 2020;**20**(1):319. DOI: 10.1186/s12893-020-00988-1

[15] Losu PU, Lal R, Gupta AK, Chaudhary P. Assessment of quality of life using EuraHS-QoL score and postoperative outcome measures following endoscopic video-assisted component separation with laparoscopic intraperitoneal onlay mesh repair in large midline ventral hernia repair. International Journal of Abdominal Wall and Hernia Surgery. 2023;**6**(4):215-221. DOI: 10.4103/ijawhs.ijawhs_9_23

[16] Tan G, Jensen MP, Thornby JI, Shanti BF. Validation of the brief pain inventory for chronic nonmalignant pain. The Journal of Pain. 2004;**5**(2):133-137. DOI: 10.1007/s00268-007-9121-4

[17] Ibrahim AA, Akindele MO, Ganiyu SO, Kaka B, Abdullahi BB, Sulaiman SK, et al. The Hausa 12-item short-form health survey (SF-12): Translation, cross-cultural adaptation and validation in mixed urban and rural Nigerian populations with chronic low back pain. Montazeri a, editor. PLoS One. 2020;**15**(5):e0232223

[18] Andresen K, Rosenberg J. Management of chronic pain after hernia repair. Journal of Pain Research. 2018;**11**:675-681. DOI: 10.2147/JPR.S127820

[19] Loos MJA, Roumen RMH, Scheltinga MRM. Classifying postherniorrhaphy pain syndromes following elective inguinal hernia repair. World Journal of Surgery. 2007;**31**(9):1760-1765

[20] Kulacoglu H. Current options in inguinal hernia repair in adult patients. Hippokratia. 2011;**15**(3):223-231

Chapter 7

The Open Abdomen: A Comprehensive Narrative Review of the Life-Threatening Condition for 2024

Svetlana Doris Brincat and Raimundas Lunevicius

Abstract

An open abdomen is a treatment option for patients with severe, life-threatening diseases or traumatic injuries. Its management poses significant challenges and involves complex clinical decisions. This chapter reviews the definitions, classifications, and treatment principles of an open abdomen, along with management strategies. The primary goal is to save the patient's life, minimize morbidity, and achieve abdominal closure, ideally through primary fascial closure. Synthetic mesh-mediated traction of fascia and laparotomy wound temporary coverage with negative pressure systems is recommended when early abdominal wall closure is impossible. If direct fascial suturing is not achievable after 2–3 attempts within 7–10 days, the fascial gap should be bridged using biological or polypropylene-reinforced biological meshes. Abdominal wall reconstruction can be performed as an alternative to mesh-mediated traction and fascial bridging for physiologically stable, uninfected patients. Incisional hernias are common after primary fascial closure and tissue bridging. Patients should be informed about it and receive appropriate counseling. A multidisciplinary approach is essential for managing open abdomen patients in hospital and outpatient settings.

Keywords: open abdomen, abdominal closure, temporary abdominal closure, definitive abdominal closure, primary fascial closure, negative pressure therapy, bridging, incisional hernia, abdominal wall reconstruction

1. Introduction

1.1 Definition

An open abdomen (OA) is a condition in which the key layer of the abdominal wall—musculofascial—is left exposed to the atmosphere by medical intention after a surgical procedure. In other words, it is a full-thickness defect within the abdominal wall formed in order to gain local and systematic therapeutic and (or) preventative effects [1].

On one hand, the practice of leaving the abdomen open after a damage-control (viz. abbreviated) surgical procedure has undeniably transformed the management of abdominal catastrophes in terms of improved survival of critically ill or injured patients [1, 2]. On the other hand, prolonged exposure of the gastrointestinal tract to the atmosphere is associated with adverse medical and surgical events, especially in low-resource settings. Therefore, all efforts (immediate, early, or delayed) should be made to restore the musculofascial anatomy of the abdominal wall or close the abdominal cavity with or without skin approximation at a physiologically acceptable time, not putting the patient at risk of abdominal compartment syndrome (ACS) [1].

The traumatic loss of the abdominal wall is a different issue. It should be viewed as one of the indications for applying temporary and (or) definitive methods to close the abdominal cavity and the wall.

1.2 Historical contributions

Several significant historical events shaped the current practice of OA management [2]. **Table 1** summarizes them [3–15].

1.3 Indications

The indications for OA are broadly categorized into physiologic, anatomic, and logistical [16].

Year	Author	Contribution
1897	McCosh	Coverage of the intestines with gauze allowing egress of peritoneal fluids. Traction to open laparotomy wound edges with two to three silkworm-gut sutures.
1940	Ogilvie	Utilization of sterilized Vaseline-coated light canvas to bridge laparotomy wounds that could not be primarily closed because of peritonitis.
1979	Steinberg	Open abdomen for patients with generalizing suppurative peritonitis.
1982	Leguit	Zipper method for temporary abdominal closure.
1983	Stone	Concept of trauma damage-control laparotomy—packing the abdominal cavity, open abdomen protecting the viscera, resuscitation in the intensive care unit, definitive repair of injuries within the next 24–72 hours.
1984	Borraez	The Bogota bag as abdominal viscera containment method: suturing a large intravenous bag to the skin edges.
1984	Kron	Open abdomen as a concept for abdominal compartment syndrome treatment.
1989	Fietsam	Treating abdominal compartment syndrome by opening the abdomen, leaving it; following abdominal aorta surgery.
1990	Ramirez	Abdominal wall component separation technique.
1990	Wittmann	Velcro adhesive sheet technique.
1991	Schein	The sandwich technique and zipper technique.
1995	Brock	Vacuum pack technique.
1997	Argenta	Negative pressure therapy.
2001	Garner	Vacuum-assisted wound closure.
2002	Miller	Vacuum-assisted fascial closure.
2008	Reimer	Dynamic retention sutures – ABRA® (abdominal approximation anchor) system.
2009	Björck	Classification of an open abdomen.

Table 1.
Historic events that transformed the management of an open abdomen.

Continuous hemodynamic instability due to severe global physiological disturbances is a physiologic indication for OA. Persistent hypotension and the components of the so-called lethal triad—acidosis (pH <7.2), hypothermia (< 34°C) and coagulopathy—are the predictors and indications of OA. Therefore, it must be borne in mind that, in critical situations, a decision to perform a damage-control abdominal surgical procedure should be made early if the lethal triad is prognosticated, as the speed of a surgical procedure may be the most important factor in the patient's complex resuscitation process and pathway [16, 17].

Anatomic indications are present when abdominal closure is impossible due to trauma or infection-related soft tissue loss or a high risk of ACS. Severe visceral or retroperitoneal oedema, loss of abdominal wall tissue, and the effects of aggressive resuscitation, such as large volumes of resuscitation fluid administered due to blood loss or septic shock, are critical factors in determining whether to close the abdominal wall or not. These conditions can lead to increased intra-abdominal pressure and complicate the abdominal wall closure, as excessive swelling or fluid retention may make it difficult to approximate the fascial edges without risking ACS. In such cases, delaying closure and opting for temporary abdominal closure techniques are necessary to ensure patient safety and resolution of edema and inflammation [16, 17].

Logistical indications for an OA are relevant for patients who require multiple abdominal surgeries to preserve the fascia. This may involve controlling hemorrhage through intraabdominal packing, managing extensive abdominal contamination by stapled resection of the injured bowel, or scheduling a second-look procedure for cases of intestinal ischemia. An emergency patient transfer between healthcare facilities within a geographical region can also necessitate using OA as a logistical measure [16, 17].

1.4 Surgery settings and patient populations

OA is a life-saving surgical intervention or standalone therapeutic procedure applicable in five critical scenarios: major trauma, intra-abdominal sepsis, vascular emergencies, acute complicated pancreatitis, and ACS. While the subsequent surgical management of OA—such as the timing and frequency of abdominal re-exploration, as well as temporary and definitive abdominal wall closure—depends on a variety of patient, injury, and disease-specific factors, some care principles remain consistent across all subpopulations. These include focused resuscitation, organ support, and nutrition management, typically provided in general or specialized critical care units [3].

1.5 Aim

Although the indications for OA have remained stable over many years, the temporary and definitive abdominal wall closure methods have significantly evolved. This narrative review of the literature has aimed to highlight the current knowledge of a patient's physiological response to an injury of any origin; to describe the management of OA; to describe temporary and definitive abdominal wall closure methods and some sequelae, such as incisional hernia; and to identify key themes that may inform future research.

1.6 Method

A literature search was conducted using three databases: PubMed, CINAHL, and Embase. This narrative review followed the SANRA instrument, the Scale for the

Assessment of Narrative Review Articles, to ensure quality [18]. The clinical scenarios and visual materials (images) are original and were selected from the individual archives of clinical practice.

2. Pathophysiology in patients with OA

The pathophysiology of OA involves a complex interplay of physiological processes that arise due to the inability to close the abdominal wall after surgery. Systemic adverse medical events include significant losses of fluids, proteins, electrolytes, micronutrients, and heat. Local adverse events such as excessive adhesions and intestinal perforations are regarded as the most critical complications associated with OA. The pathophysiological effects are classified into two broad phases [19].

2.1 Phase 1

During the initial phase of damage-control surgery—focused on resuscitation and stabilization of physiology—patients often experience severe metabolic imbalances due to cardiovascular instability, hemorrhage, sepsis, systemic inflammatory response, and coagulation disorders resulting from the primary injury. Consequently, the initial surgery should be concise, ideally lasting 30 to 40 minutes or less, utilizing a temporary abdominal closure technique to facilitate the patient's swift transfer to the intensive care unit to stabilize the physiological systems while mitigating the adverse effects of an OA [19].

A second surgery is typically required within 24–48 hours to remove surgical packs, achieve definitive surgical hemostasis, restore bowel continuity, assess organ viability, establish enteric diversions, or debride necrotic or infected tissue. In cases of severe intra-abdominal infections, such as infected necrotizing pancreatitis, open debridement every 48 hours may be necessary when minimally invasive methods of treatment cannot be applied [19].

During this phase, the peritoneal cavity produces a substantial volume of cytokine-rich fluid, which can have harmful systemic effects and exacerbate metabolic disturbances [19]. The use of negative-pressure abdominal wound therapy systems, for example, the 3 M™ AbThera™ Negative Pressure Wound Therapy, is crucial to prevent the absorption of these endogenous toxins.

Efforts should be made to achieve a definitive fascial closure of the musculofascial layer of the abdominal wall by the end of the first phase of damage control surgery. At this stage of the disease, patients typically exhibit improved hemodynamic stability and metabolic recovery, and tissue edema is often reduced enough to allow for safe abdominal wall closure without excessive tension. Concurrently, natural wound-healing processes begin, forming adhesions between the intestines, omentum, and parietal peritoneum. Consequently, laparotomy wound edges begin to contract due to lateral retraction of the abdominal muscles.

2.2 Phase 2

The second phase occurs when no further intra-abdominal procedures are required, but the abdominal wall cannot yet be closed due to tissue swelling. If the fascia remains open at the end of this phase, it is necessary to cover the wound using skin-only methods, either through primary closure or partial-thickness skin grafts.

If fascial closure is not achieved within 7 days (an 8–10-day term is also acceptable in extraordinary circumstances), a "frozen visceral sac" develops. This involves visceral structures adhering to the peritoneal gutters, with lateralization of the fascial edges, leading to a widened wound, loss of domain, and the inability to close the fascia primarily [19]. When a "frozen visceral sac" is apparent or significant edema of the bowel, abdominal wall, or retroperitoneal tissues persists, making tension-free closure impossible, alternative techniques for abdominal cavity closure should be considered. The interval between skin coverage and the final abdominal wall reconstruction may represent the third phase [20].

Primary abdominal wall closure by layer is achieved in 34–74% of patients. For those unable to achieve this outcome, the risk of developing incisional hernias significantly increases [20].

2.3 Complications of OA: Bowel perforation and enteroatmospheric fistula

Increased likelihood of enteroatmospheric fistula (EAF) formation, particularly when the abdominal wall cannot be closed within 1 week, is a well-documented risk of an OA. Bowel perforation is one of the most feared complications in OA, as the bowel is vulnerable to adverse conditions such as desiccation, mechanical shearing during dressing changes, and movement against the covering sheath. Injuries to the bowel serosa further heighten the risk of perforations. When these perforations are not covered by viable, well-perfused tissue and are exposed within the wound, they result in EAF, which can develop in 20% of patients with OAs [21]. It is important to note the lowest EAF rate is in the trauma patient population and the highest rate (approximately 50%) in patients with infected pancreatic necrosis [19, 22].

2.4 Fistula risk mitigation

Given the high morbidity risk associated with OA, surgeons must take steps to mitigate intestinal complications. It is important to remember that the primary goal of managing patients with abdominal catastrophes is to save lives with minimal exposure to harm; hernia prevention is a task of secondary importance in these difficult situations. For instance, continuing mesh-mediated traction beyond 8 to 10 days (in more than 2–3 attempts) is doubtful surgical practice. Instead, surgeons should consider alternatives like intraperitoneal bridging techniques using transfascial sutures for biological mesh fixation to the parietal peritoneum of the abdominal wall. The use of biological matrix-based hernia meshes to cover visceral organs and prevent EAF—regardless of whether skin closure is possible—has been re-emphasized in recent years. Polypropylene mesh, when used for bridge repair of the OA, is associated with high rates of EAF formation and is, therefore, not recommended for these procedures [22, 23].

3. Classification of an OA

A classification finalized in 2016, resulting from the first version of the OA classification and the update from the World Society of the Abdominal Compartment

Class	Description
1	No adherence between bowel and abdominal wall or fixity (i.e., lateralization) of the abdominal wall
1A	Clean tissues, open abdomen
1B	Contaminated tissues, open abdomen
1C	Enteric leak*
2	Developing adherence (fixity) between bowel and abdominal wall
2A	Clean
2B	Contaminated
2C	Enteric leak*
3	Frozen (i.e., fixed, lateralized) abdomen
3A	Clean
3B	Contaminated
4	Enteroatmospheric fistula**

*****An enteric leak controlled by closure, exteriorization into a stoma, or a permanent enterocutaneous fistula should be classed as 1A or 2A.*
***Permanent enteric leak into the open abdomen associated with granulation tissue.*

Table 2.
Classification of an open abdomen.

Syndrome, is recommended for use (**Table 2**) [3, 15, 21, 24]. It uniformizes OA reporting standards, facilitates comparisons across patient cohorts, and helps define the goals of various treatment modalities and strategies.

4. Temporary closure of the abdomen

Temporary abdominal closure is often required after a damage-control procedure (see 1.3. Indications) as it reduces postoperative morbidity, hence increasing survival chance. In ideal circumstances, temporary abdominal closure should provide atraumatic coverage for the exposed abdominal organs using materials that have a low adhesive potential to the visceral peritoneum, prevent ACS, minimize the loss of physiological fluids and heat, facilitate easy re-entry into the abdomen, and enhance the likelihood of delayed primary abdominal wall closure [19]. As shown in **Table 3**, the methods for temporal abdominal closure can be broadly grouped into the following categories [25, 26].

4.1 Skin-only closure techniques

These are the most straightforward techniques to cover the abdominal cavity, leaving the linea alba or fascial-muscular layer open. They are typically executed using towel clips, a running monofilament suture, or surgical clips. The 1 cm rule should be followed when these techniques are employed. Towel clips are placed on the skin about 1 cm apart and 1 cm away from each other. Positioning the handles of all the towel clips toward the center allows for easier coverage of these clips with an adhesive plastic or any other drape. A similar distance (1 cm) should be kept for a running suture. Surgical skin clips, as the alternative to continuous suture, should also be placed approximately 1 cm away from each other [25].

Method	Description	Characteristics
Skin only closure		
Continuous suture	Skin provides abdominal wall stability and containment	↑ Evisceration risk ↑ Abdominal compartment syndrome ↑ Infection risk
Towel clips		
Patch closure		
Home-made materials		
Packing and dressings	Placing non adherent wet swabs or hydrophilic dressings directly on top of abdominal viscera	↑ Evisceration risk ↑ Fluid and protein loss ↑ Fistulization risk
Bogota bag	Use of sterile plastic bag	Easily accessible Transparent Inert Peritoneal fluid not evacuated
Wittmann patch	Patch sutured to fascia and tightened every 24–48 hours	↑ Fascial trauma and necrosis, as it requires suturing to fascia ↑ Risk incisional hernia No evacuation of peritoneal fluid Costly
Zipper closure	Sheet with a sterilized zipper sutured with the fascial edges	↑ Risk of trauma of underlying abdominal viscera from opening and closing the zipper
Commercial mesh utilization		
Synthetic	Fixation to fascial edges. Intraperitoneal fixation using transfascial sutures.	↑Infection risk using synthetic meshes ↑ Fistulization risk with synthetic mesh ↑Cost of biological mesh
Biological		
Reinforced biological matrix		
Vacuum-assisted closure, negative pressure therapy (NPT)		
Alone*	Utilizes the principles of reverse tissue expansion to promote tissue growth and facilitate wound closure.	↑ Local blood perfusion and nutrient delivery to the wound ↑ Wound vascularity ↑ Granulation tissue ↑ Cell proliferation and angiogenesis ↓ Bowel oedema ↓ Wound contamination ↓ Frequent dressing change
Combined with patch closure		
Combined with mediated fascia traction		
Dynamic retention sutures		
Alone (no additional devices)**	Plastic tubes inserted through the skin across the abdominal defect and are attached to the skin on both sides of the wound by button anchors.	Reliable coverage with adequate abdominal wall opposition. Gradual elimination of intrabdominal hypertension.
Combined with NPT		

**AbThera™, VAC (vacuum-assisted wound closure), as the examples.*
***ABRA®, abdominal re-approximation anchor device, as an example.*

Table 3.
Systemization of the methods for temporary abdominal closure.

It is a quick, cost-effective, and accessible method, especially pertinent in low-resource settings. Physiologically, this approach keeps the abdominal contents below the fascia, reducing heat and fluid loss. Anatomically, the connections between the skin, subcutaneous tissue, and underlying muscles may help prevent loss of domain when only the skin is closed. According to some reports [20], skin-only temporal abdominal wall closure techniques are associated with a high fascial closure rate of 82% and a moderate (6%) risk of EAF.

It is important to note that the applicability of this method is restricted because of the skin's low bursting pressure and the limited ability of the approximated skin to stretch in response to worsening visceral edema. Therefore, the scientific literature recommend abandoning the skin-only closure technique when other resources are available [27]. The arguments against this technique include its inability to control abdominal effluents, interference with radiographic imaging when towel clips are used, a high incidence of ACS ranging from 13 to 36%, failure to prevent loss of domain, a high risk of evisceration, and frequent skin injury and loss [28]. However, these recommendations should be interpreted cautiously as they were derived from retrospective, highly heterogeneous studies, many of which did not include essential clinical outcomes.

Available knowledge on managing OA suggests that decision-making in emergency surgery should be highly individual and mostly dependent on the patient's factors, injury origin and grade, prognosis, and further surgical action planning. For example, the increased intra-abdominal pressure associated with skin-only closure may aid hemostasis in patients experiencing ongoing bleeding after damage-control laparotomy. Preliminary data from the International Register of OA suggest that skin-only closure, as well as Bogota bags, is linked to higher rates of primary fascial closure and lower mortality in trauma patients compared to negative pressure therapy (NPT) dressing systems [20]. However, as pointed out earlier, these findings should be interpreted cautiously.

The authors of this chapter prefer a running suture if a decision is made to use one of the skin-only closure techniques. Trauma damage-control laparotomy with perihepatic packing and drainage is a realistic scenario and example. Trauma damage-control laparotomy with splenectomy and left subphrenic space packing is another scenario and example. Furthermore, temporary closure of linea alba and skin is also a good option when relaparotomy is planned within the next 24–48 hours.

4.2 Patch closure

Patch-based techniques for temporary abdominal closure create a barrier between the peritoneum and the external environment, reducing fluid and heat loss. However, compared to vacuum closure techniques, patch methods are less effective at removing peritoneal fluid, which is particularly crucial for patients undergoing temporary abdominal closure due to intra-abdominal sepsis. Additionally, while patch closure allows some expansion of the intra-abdominal contents beyond their normal anatomical boundaries, this expansion is limited to the patch's fixed size, making it possible for ACS to develop [20, 23].

4.2.1 Packing and dressings

Covering the abdominal contents with large swabs or surgical drapes without suturing these materials to the fascia is acceptable in difficult surgical circumstances when there are no other options or time. The adhesive dressing perforated at a few sites is used to fix the swabs or drapes to the skin. This method is advantageous due to its simplicity, availability, quick application, and low cost. Relook surgery needs to be done within the next 12–24 hours. Other methods of temporary abdominal closure should be considered and planned before surgical re-exploration of the abdominal cavity [29].

4.2.1.1 Scenario 1, emergency general surgery setting

A female patient in her 40s presented to the accident and emergency department with a septic shock secondary to a perforated left-sided colon. Emergency midline laparotomy revealed perforated diverticulitis of the middle portion of the sigmoid colon, large pericolic abscess cavity, and generalizing peritonitis. Cardiac peri-arrest occurred. GIA Auto Suture staplers with DST series technology were used to resect the perforated sigmoid colon. After washing out the abdominal cavity, the left lower area of the abdominal cavity was packed, and the laparotomy wound and visceral contents were covered by 18 × 18 cm and 12 × 12 cm swabs. A large adhesive bandage was used to dress the laparotomy wound. As the patient's physiological condition was grossly unstable, and circumstances in the operating theater were extraordinary, applying a commercial intraabdominal negative pressure device (AbThera™) was not considered. After damage-control surgery, the multiorgan dysfunction and disseminated intravascular coagulopathy progressed rapidly within hours in the intensive care unit. Re-exploration of the abdominal cavity and amputation of the ischemic leg were discussed a few times as a possibility.

4.2.1.2 Scenario 2, elective hernia surgery setting

A male patient in his 70s presented to the day surgery center for incisional moderate-size irreducible hernia repair. During the first phase of laparoscopic surgery (hostile abdomen and dense adhesions all over the peritoneal cavity documented), sudden profuse arterial bleeding occurred, resulting in gross hemodynamic instability. The shared decision-making process for surgical and anesthetist teams was activated immediately. The control (suture-ligation) of the injured vessels of the great omentum and mesentery of the colon was achieved after immediate laparotomy. Stapled resection of an ischemic transverse colon without colostomy formation, splenectomy, and primary repair of the small intestine were the next necessary surgical actions. The abdominal cavity, including the left subphrenic space, was packed using 18 × 18 cm swabs. An adhesive bandage was used to dress the laparotomy wound (i.e., open abdomen). The first re-exploration of the abdominal cavity was carried out after 24 hours. A transverse colostomy was formed, and definitive tension-free closure of the abdominal cavity by layer was achieved. Loop polydioxanone (PDS) size 1 sutures were utilized for fascial closure. The patient survived.

4.2.2 Bogota bag

The "Bogota bag" is a plastic bag sutured to the skin. It involves using an intravenous bag to cover the abdominal viscera. Following the initial surgical actions, a sterilized, soft 3-liter intravenous bag is cut into an oval shape and attached to the skin edges of the wound using a continuous monofilament suture. Sterile, antibiotic-soaked towels are placed over the bag and then covered with an iodine-impregnated adhesive plastic drape. The dressing is changed every 24 hours in the operating theater or intensive care unit [25, 30–32].

Translucent patch material allows the examination of intra-abdominal contents without reopening the abdominal cavity. However, it has significant limitations. One is the difficulty in controlling high-volume fluid secretions from the abdomen, and another is the lack of promotion of direct primary closure [20, 25].

The use of a Bogota bag is linked to a high incidence of postoperative morbidity and delayed complications. In a series of 86 patients, Manterola et al. [30] found that the most common reason for the relaparotomy followed by a laparostomy using the Bogota bag was intra-abdominal sepsis (60%). The primary fascial closure rate was 39%, with an in-hospital mortality rate of 12%. Within a 48-month follow-up period, ventral hernia developed in 60% of these patients.

Notably, primary fascial closure rates reported in the literature vary widely from 12–82%. The explanation that the absence of negative pressure might account for the reported low incidence of EAF (ranging from 0 to 14.4%) is unconvincing.

Surgical drapes fixed to the skin can be used instead of intravenous fluid bags when a Bogota bag cannot be made in operating theaters or critical circumstances [25].

4.2.3 Wittmann patch

In 1990, Wittman et al. introduced Velcro-like material for temporary abdominal closure in patients with intra-abdominal sepsis. This technique involves suturing two sheets of material to the abdominal fascia, which engage with each other to keep the abdomen closed. Re-entry is facilitated by separating the sheets every 24–48 hours, which can be sequentially advanced and trimmed to aid fascial closure. At the time of definitive closure, the sheets are removed [33]. The Wittman patch achieves primary fascial closure in 66–100% of cases, with an EAF incidence ranging from 0 to 42%. Long-term follow-up data show no incidence of incisional hernia, making this treatment safe and effective. Despite its effectiveness, the Wittman patch is costly, which limits its use. The inability to drain intraperitoneal fluid is another disadvantage of the Wittman patch [20, 33].

4.2.4 Zipper closure

Zipper closure uses a sterile zipper sutured to the fascia to cover the abdominal organs and tissues [34, 35]. Though its use declined, recent studies report primary fascial closure rates of 50–100% [36, 37]. This technique is inexpensive and straightforward to implement. However, it fell out of favor due to several drawbacks, such as the potential for increased intra-abdominal pressure, the inability to drain intra-abdominal fluids, and the difficulty in assessing intra-abdominal contents without reopening the abdomen [20, 36].

4.2.5 Mesh utilization

For the management of OA, meshes can be used to bridge and close the fascial defect or for abdominal wall reconstruction.

Synthetic mesh-based, tension-free temporary abdominal closure was introduced in the 1980s to facilitate the re-exploration of the abdominal cavity. The rationale for using synthetic mesh for temporary abdominal closure is as follows: when sutured to the fascial edges, the mesh protects intra-abdominal and abdominal wall tissues from damage caused by repeated surgical procedures, prevents lateral retraction of the fascia, and facilitates the operation to close the abdominal fascia. The mesh or sheet can be cut in the center during the re-exploration of the abdominal cavity and then re-sutured to bring the two edges together. This procedure is often combined with NPT to enhance primary fascial closure of the abdominal wall [25]. The mesh can also be removed during re-operation, and if fascial closure is not achieved initially, it can be trimmed and re-apposed to bring the fascial edges closer [33].

Various mesh types have been used. Complications such as mesh infection, hernia, mesh extrusion, and EAF are common. Polypropylene mesh has fallen out of favor due to a high risk of EAF, occurring in up to 34% of cases. Polytetrafluoroethylene (PTFE) mesh, while less adherent to the bowel, is prone to bacterial colonization, increasing infection risk [20, 37, 38]. Biodegradable meshes made from synthetic polymers (polyglactin or polyglycolic acid) show better outcomes, with lower fistula rates (5–11%) than polypropylene [23]. These meshes promote granulation tissue formation, facilitating skin grafting when primary fascial closure is impossible.

The advent of biological and absorbable synthetic meshes has introduced a viable alternative to traditional options. These meshes, sourced from biologic materials (such as human, bovine, porcine, or ovine) or absorbable synthetic components, are designed to integrate with native tissue while offering resistance to infection. A key advantage promoted for biologic meshes is their suitability for use in contaminated environments, reducing the risk of infection and the need for explantation. Biological meshes support vascular ingrowth—cross-linked ones less, not-crossed-linked ones more—enabling the host immune system to combat infections, unlike synthetic meshes, which lack this capability [33, 39, 40].

Reinforced biological matrix meshes represent a new generation of meshes that blend biological and synthetic materials. These meshes are engineered to minimize foreign body reactions while promoting tissue remodeling. They consist of layers of biological material interwoven with polymer using a specialized lock-stitch pattern. The inclusion of polymer enhances strength, improves handling, and optimizes load-sharing capabilities. This combination increases the mesh's durability, handling ease, and ability to distribute forces during stretching.

Additionally, microchannels within the mesh facilitate fluid transfer, enabling rapid absorption of wound fluids and blood during implantation. These channels also support cellular infiltration and migration, essential for functional tissue remodeling during healing. Overall, reinforced biological matrix meshes are designed to handle and suture easily [33, 40].

4.2.5.1 Bridging mesh

The mesh is fixed to the abdominal wall fascia using interrupted or continuous sutures, typically with polypropylene or polydioxanone to the fascial edges. As an alternative to this method, transfascial intraperitoneal fixation of mesh—using individual U-shape sutures—can be performed approximately 3–5 cm away from the fascial edges. If skin closure is impossible due to edema or concerns about abscess formation, the mesh can be covered with a moist dressing that is changed daily, or a wound VAC can be applied over the mesh and changed every 5–7 days. The mesh fascia anatomical relationship is checked during each dressing change, as its laxity may occur when visceral edema subsides. If laxity is detected, a synthetic absorbable mesh can be carefully folded at the midline using primary fascial closure in the operating room.

On the other hand, if granulation tissue forms before the fascial edges can be approximated, a skin graft may be applied over the mesh, applicable to both biological and synthetic absorbable meshes. Skin graft removal and primary fascial closure or abdominal wall reconstruction can be scheduled 6 to 12 months later [17, 19].

4.3 Vacuum-assisted closure: Negative pressure therapy

4.3.1 Barker's vacuum-packing technique

This approach is cost-effective. It consists of a fenestrated, nonadherent sterile nylon sheet placed over the viscera as a protective barrier, effectively preventing adhesion formation. While bowel loops may adhere to each other, the area between the bowel and the abdominal wall stays clear, allowing the abdominal wall to remain mobile. This sheet is then covered with moist surgical towels or gauze as a wound filter. Two drains are placed over the towels or gauze. The wound is then sealed with an adhesive occlusive dressing to create an airtight seal, with the drains connected to a negative pressure-generating device for continuous suction at 100–150 mmHg (usually at 125 mmHg). Barker et al. reported 68.1% primary fascial closure, 5% EAF, and 1.2% ACS rates [19, 20, 41].

4.3.2 Commercial negative pressure systems

Commercial negative pressure systems like VAC and AbThera™ use polyurethane sponges under a fenestrated polyethylene sheet, covered with an adhesive dressing to create a seal.

VAC is an advanced negative pressure dressing system that consists of a polyurethane foam covered with a protected, fenestrated, non-adherent layer, connected by a tube to a canister and computerized pump. This system prevents adhesions between the bowel and the anterior abdominal wall, facilitates easy abdominal re-exploration, and maintains tension on the fascia [20].

AbThera™ is a device featuring a visceral protective layer made of polyurethane foam with six radiating foam extensions enveloped in a polyethylene sheet with small fenestrations. This layer is placed in the abdominal cavity beneath the abdominal wall to protect the bowel, extending into the paracolic gutters and pelvis. It effectively removes peritoneal fluid. The polyurethane foam is positioned between the incisional margins and covered with a sterile adhesive drape. A small section of the adhesive drape and underlying sponge is excised, and an interface pad with a tubing system is applied over the defect and connected to a pump and canister to collect fluids. Dressing changes are typically performed every 48–72 hours (**Figure 1**) [42].

These modern devices offer several advantages over older systems like the Barker's Vacuum Pack. They allow for higher negative pressure from the periphery to the center, improving the efficacy of removing intra-abdominal toxins, bacteria-rich fluids, and pro-inflammatory cytokines (**Table 3**). These devices are also easier to manage for nursing staff, reduce visceral edema, and maintain the tension between the muscular edges [20].

In a study by Cheatham [43], the 30-day primary fascial closure rate was approximately 70% in the AbThera™ group compared to 51% in the Barker group ($p = 0.03$), with lower mortality in the AbThera™ group (14% for AbThera™ group and 30% for Barker group, $p = 0.01$). The latter was further confirmed in the RCT by Kirkpatrick et al. [44], who reported that the AbThera™ group had a lower 90-day mortality rate compared to the Barker vacuum-packing group (21.7% for AbThera™ group *versus* 50.0% for the Barker group, $p = 0.04$) of primary fascial closure.

It is important to note that these systems can be used for patients with coagulation disorders and diffuse oozing from abdominal organs and tissues to cover abdominal viscera and achieve temporary abdominal closure without activating negative pressure.

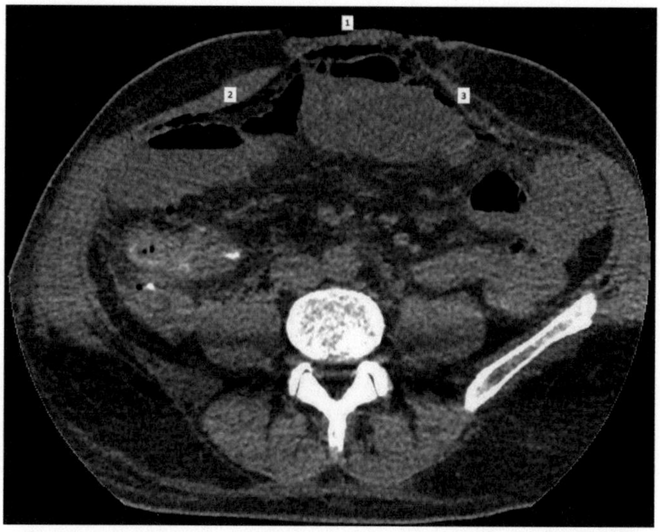

Figure 1.
Radiological appearances of the abdominal wall after the temporary closure of the abdomen utilizing a commercial device with negative pressure therapy; a computed tomography scan was performed on the 1st day after the first re-exploration of the abdominal cavity. Digits: 1 –3M™ AbThera™ advanced open abdomen dressing system component—3M™ SensaT.R.A.C.™ Pad. 2 – right rectus abdominis muscle. 3 – left rectus abdominis muscle. Synopsis of the case: Damage control midline laparotomy and stapled ischemic small bowel (ileum) resection were performed for a critically unwell patient whose past surgical history included right hemicolectomy with primary anastomosis. The endovascular aortic aneurysm repair was followed by the first abdominal cavity re-exploration and resection of the ischemic ileocolic segment in 10–12 hours. During both operations, 3M™ AbThera™ advanced open abdomen dressing system with active negative pressure therapy was utilized for temporary abdominal wall closure.

5. Dynamic retention sutures: An abdominal approximation anchor, ABRA®

The ABRA® system facilitates the approximation of wound and muscle edges through dynamic traction exerted by transfascial elastomers. This technique involves inserting plastic tubes through all abdominal wall layers, positioned 1 cm away from the fascial edge and secured with an adhesive button. Negative pressure techniques can also be applied to the defect during margin re-approximation to drain intra-abdominal fluids. The tubes are usually adjusted every 24–36 hours by pulling them from both sides of the defect to gradually achieve a final approximation of the abdominal wall. When the fascial edges are within 1 cm, the ABRA® system can be removed, and the surgical incision—fascia or muscular-fascial layer and skin—can be closed. Thus, this method can be used for temporary and definitive abdominal wall closures [29, 33].

It is not a straightforward method to implement. In addition, the disadvantages of this method include the risk of developing ACS and an increased likelihood of EAF due to tube pressure on the intestinal tract [20, 29].

6. Re-exploration before definitive closure

The indications for re-exploring an OA differ between non-trauma and trauma patients. For non-trauma patients, the indications for re-exploration are less clear and often include the need to continue damage control management due to the inability to control the source of infection, the necessity to reassess bowel vascularization, or rising concerns about the possibility of ACS. Generally, if a patient fails to show improvement, it may be due to an intra-abdominal issue.

There is no definitive data on the optimal timing for re-operation in OA patients. However, it is generally recommended that patients with an OA should be re-explored within 24–72 hours after the initial or any subsequent surgical intervention. Data on trauma patients indicate that delaying re-exploration beyond the first 24 hours post-initial operation decreases the primary fascial closure rate by 1.1% per hour. Also, patients who undergo their first re-operation after 48 hours experience higher complication rates [17, 23].

7. Definitive closure of the abdominal wall

Early abdominal closure is the primary aim of managing patients with an OA, as the complication rate significantly increases beyond 2 weeks after initial damage-control surgery. The success largely depends on two critical factors: the temporary abdominal closure techniques employed and the patient's postoperative stabilization in the critical care unit.

7.1 Timing

Ensuring optimal physiologic support post-surgery in the intensive care unit is essential for facilitating timely and effective abdominal wall closure. Also, ruling out ongoing intraabdominal issues, such as persistent or new infections, bowel ischemia, biliary or intestinal leaks, or bleeding, is key for successful definitive abdominal wall closure. It is essential to weigh the benefits of early abdominal wall closure against the potential risks of managing an OA.

Fascial closure within the first 7 days following the first operation is defined as early; sooner is better if the patient's condition and surrounding circumstances allow. Typically, it occurs on postoperative days 4–7, though an 8–10-day window is also acceptable. However, unlike trauma patients, those with abdominal sepsis tend to have lower rates of early fascial closure, even with the use of mesh-mediated fascial traction [17].

7.2 Definitive closure techniques

As shown in **Table 4**, definitive abdominal closure methods can be classified into four broad categories: primary fascial closure, bridging, component separation, and dynamic retention sutures. They can be used as a single surgical treatment option or in combination [17, 25, 29].

7.2.1 Fascial closure

7.2.1.1 Primary fascial closure

For most patients, definitive abdominal fascia closure is typically achieved during a second operation within 24 to 48 hours of the initial surgery. A slowly absorbable

Method	Characteristics: description, indication, benefits, risks
Fascial closure Primary Dynamic mesh-mediated primary Alone; no additional devices Combined with NPT Commercial-device traction	Fascial closure can be performed using long-term absorbable monofilament sutures. Meshes can be used to aid fascial closure. Mesh mediated-fascial traction can occur in 2–3 attempts. It can be used alone with no additional devices when NPT systems are unavailable. When combined with NPT, it provides the highest primary fascial closure rates. Commercial-device traction (Fasciotens®Abdomen) requires adequate patient selection.
Bridging Direct, fascia edge to mesh edge, NPT Intraperitoneal transfascial, NPT	Biological permanent prosthetic meshes are the best choice for abdominal wall fascia bridging of any size. Two principles for bridging abdominal fascia: (1) suturing the mesh to the fascia edges; (2) transfascial intraperitoneal fixation of the mesh using individual 'U' form sutures (Section 4.2.5.1.).
Component separation Retro-muscular No TAR Extension to TAR Anterior component separation	Abdominal component separation techniques—posterior such as retro-muscular Rives-Stoppa type, transverse abdominis release, and anterior, or a combination of them—should ideally be considered as an elective procedure for ventral hernia repair. However, in the context of OA, component separation should be applied in carefully selected patients after primary vascular or parenchymal organ trauma surgery.
Dynamic retention sutures Alone (no additional devices) Combined with NPT	ABRA® can be used alone or combined with NPT. It can also be used for temporary closure and definitive abdominal closure. Dynamic retention sutures may be painful and uncomfortable, resulting in unsightly scarring and ulcerations, so reasonable tension should be applied.

Abbreviations: NPT, negative pressure therapy. TAR, transversus abdominis release. ABRA®, abdominal re-approximation anchor device.
Explanation: Fasciotens®Abdomen is a device that stretches the fascia perpendicularly during surgery to achieve a primary tension-free abdominal closure.

Table 4.
Classification of the methods for definitive abdominal closure for patients with OA.

monofilament suture, such as polydioxanone (PDS), is recommended for this procedure (**Figure 2**). Since these surgeries occur in an emergency general surgery setting, the guidelines for abdominal wall closure in elective procedures—such as those from the European and American Hernia Societies—are inapplicable to patients with an OA [45, 46]. We recommend using two loop-PDS size 1 sutures to approximate the fascia. In cases where tension makes the approximation difficult, alternative techniques should be considered, including hernia mesh-mediated closure, bridging, dynamic retention sutures, component separation, and, when appropriate, the application of NPT devices.

7.2.1.2 Hernia mesh-mediated closure

Section 4.2.5. describes the essence of hernia mesh-mediated closure during temporary abdominal closure—two or three efforts within seven (but no more than 10 in exceptional cases) days. Primary fascial closure should be reliable. Incorrect interpretation of the European Hernia Society abdominal closure guidelines—2-0 PDS continuous small bite suture—can have catastrophic consequences associated with repeatedly burst abdomen [46].

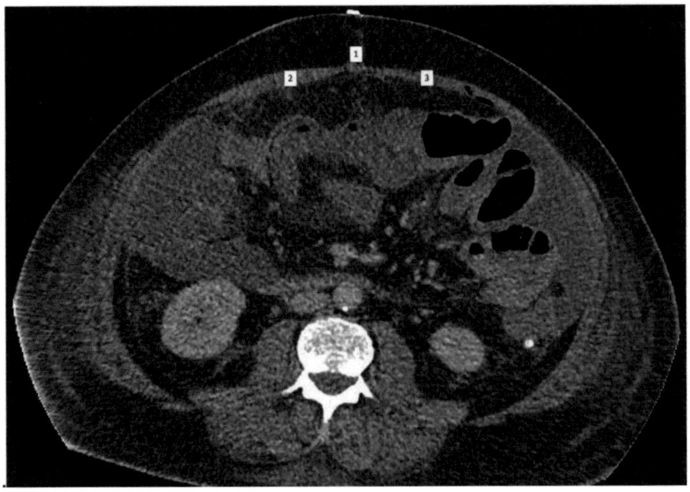

Figure 2.
Satisfactory appearances of the anterior abdominal wall radiological anatomy after definitive abdominal wall closure; a computed tomography scan was performed on the 5th day after the first re-exploration of the abdominal cavity. Primary closure of the abdominal wall was achieved—linea alba was approximated using loop-PDS (polydioxanone) size 1 continuous suture; the skin was closed using metallic clips. Digits: 1 – linea alba. 2 – right rectus abdominis muscle. 3 – left rectus abdominis muscle. Synopsis of the case: Damage control midline laparotomy was performed for a critically unwell patient. Fecal contamination of the entire peritoneal cavity secondary to perforated gangrenous caecum associated with obstructive sigmoid colon cancer was the cause of the septic shock. Multiple left hemiliver metastases were palpated. A stapled right hemicolectomy was performed just. Notably, 12 liters of saline were utilized to wash the abdominal cavity. 3M™ AbThera™ advanced open abdomen dressing system incorporating negative pressure therapy was used for temporal abdominal closure. Re-exploration of the abdomen, end ileostomy, mucus transverse colon fistula formation, and abdominal wall closure by layers were formed after 48 hours of stay in the critical care unit. The patient survived.

7.2.1.3 Commercial device-mediated intraoperative ultrashort-term traction

The Fasciotens®Abdomen device employs controlled vertical traction to prevent abdominal wall musculature from retracting while gradually and precisely stretching the abdominal wall. The Fasciotens®Abdomen system includes a stand and a thread retainer that is suspended over the abdomen during the procedure. Six sutures are attached to the fascial edges and secured to the thread retainer with fixing clips, maintaining consistent tension. The traction force applied to the abdominal wall or fascia can be fine-tuned using a screw mechanism [47].

The evidence for Fasciotens®Abdomen is limited, with data from non-comparative observational studies and case reports involving a small number of patients. In a retrospective multicenter study by Fung et al. involving 20 patients with an OA, it was observed that 48 hours after applying Fasciotens®Abdomen, the average fascial distance substantially decreased to allow for definitive fascial closure [48].

Studies on Fasciotens®Abdomen for definitive closure of an OA have not been performed in the UK [49]. Significant side effects graded as Clavien-Dindo 4B were observed within the small empirical case series (unpublished data).

7.2.2 Bridging

When a tension-free approximation of the fascia is impossible, the remaining gap must be bridged with the mesh within 7 days. Synthetic, non-absorbable meshes, such as polypropylene, should be avoided due to the increased risk of infection, intestinal erosion, and fistula formation. Instead, biological permanent meshes are preferred for bridging defects of any size [17].

Although there is continuing debate about whether cross-linked or non-cross-linked collagen meshes should be used for this purpose, our position, based on practical experience, is that non-cross-linked collagen meshes are the first choice. These meshes integrate more effectively into surrounding tissues due to enhanced revascularization, reducing fibrosis.

Two primary techniques are used for bridging the musculofascial layer of the abdominal wall. The first one involves suturing the mesh to the edges of the fascia. The second technique (recommended) is a transfascial intraperitoneal fixation of the mesh, securing it 3–5 cm from the fascial defect using individual polydioxanone (i.e., PDS) "U" shape sutures. While closing the skin and placing a negative pressure drain is ideal (**Figure 3**), this is not always feasible. In such cases, vacuum-assisted VAC® dressings are a suitable alternative to cover the bridging mesh, creating an optimal environment for wound granulation and secondary intention healing (**Figures 4–7**). Even when the skin is closed, as shown in **Figure 3**, negative pressure dressings should be applied. These dressings are commercially available, cost-effective, and accessible to healthcare facilities. 3M™ Prevena™ incision management system is one of them.

Once granulation tissue forms and appears healthy, it is advisable to consult plastic surgeons, particularly for patients with extensive thoracoabdominal defects. The granulated wound can then be covered by subcutaneous flaps on either side, and the skin can be closed in the midline. A split-thickness skin graft is another option when the abdominal wall defect is large.

7.2.3 Abdominal wall component separation

An alternative approach to closing an OA involves acute abdominal wall reconstruction using component separation techniques. Ramirez [7] introduced an anterior component separation method for repairing large abdominal wall fascial defects as

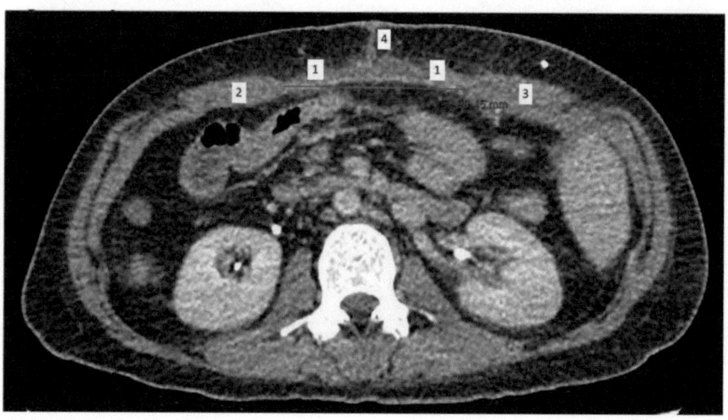

Figure 3.
Definitive abdominal closure: early bridging with delayed skin closure. Digits: 1 – Ovitex® 2S–P reinformed tissue matrix; the distance between recti muscles is 9.45 cm. 2 – right rectus abdominis muscle. 3 – left rectus abdominis muscle. 4 – skin. The summary of the surgical events and a long-term plan: (1) 3M™ AbThera™ advanced open abdomen dressing system for temporary closure of contaminated abdomen after elective intestinal surgery was performed; (2) After 48 hours, transfascial intraperitoneal fixation of Ovitex® 2S–P reinformed tissue matrix (25 × 40 cm mesh utilized; trimmed to 36 × 17 cm) and negative pressure VAC® system for abdominal closure after 48 hours were utilized; (3) Skin closure after mobilizing skin flaps bilaterally on day 10. The long-term plan is to review the patient in the abdominal wall reconstruction clinic in 12 months.

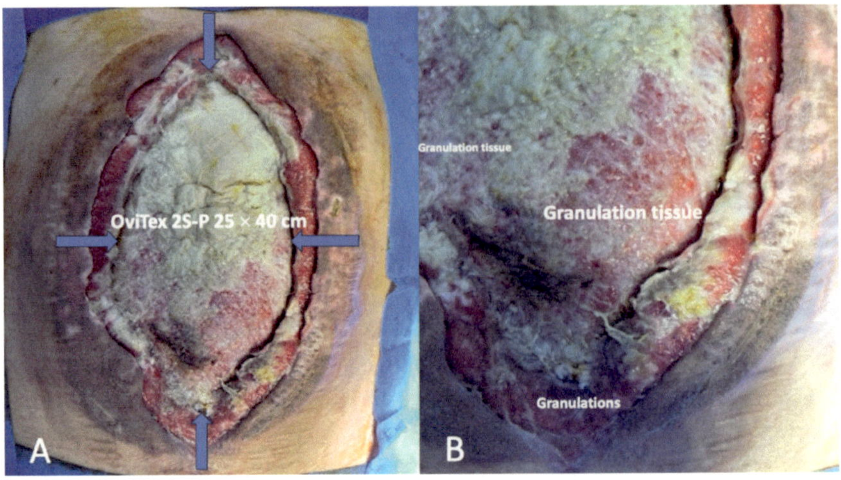

Figure 4.
Appearance of the abdominal wall on the 14th postoperative day after transfascial intraperitoneal fixation of Ovitex® 2S–P reinformed tissue matrix of 25 × 40 cm size for abdominal closure. Explanation: Ovitex® 2S–P reinformed tissue matrix is an 8-layer, not-cross-linked biological mesh with two smooth (2S) sides. The mesh matrix is produced from ovine rumen tissue and reinforced by interwoven polypropylene sutures (permanent synthetic material, 6%). The biological matrix to permanent synthetic material (polypropylene) ratio is 94 to 6. Theoretically, the patient's body remodels the biological component of this mesh into a functional collagen layer. Polypropylene holds the biological layers together and strengthens the early healing phase. However, in the event of local mesh infection—a common phenomenon managing patients with open abdomen—the biological component of the mesh gradually disintegrates, granulation tissue replaces it, and the polymer remains in situ.

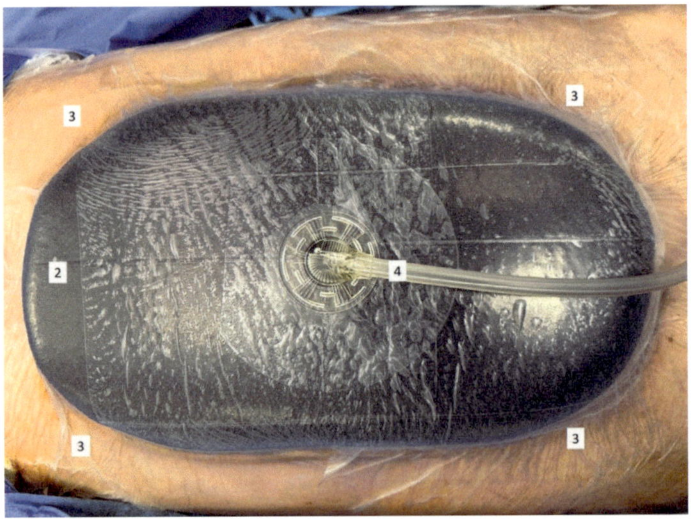

Figure 5.
Postoperative day 14th after transfascial intraperitoneal placement and fixation of an Ovitex® 2S–P reinformed tissue matrix of 25 × 40 cm size for abdominal closure: the appearance of the abdominal wall after VAC ® Granufoam™ dressing change, before activation of KSI VAC negative pressure wound system pump, 125 mm Hg. The components of the system are as follows: 1. Soft silicone wound contact layer – Silflex (Silfix® technology, Advancis Medical), covering the wound fully (invisible in the figure). 2. VAC ® Granufoam™ dressing change, medium, featuring Sensa. RAC™ technology. 3. Adhesive films covering Granufoam™ and surrounding skin (they seal the wound). 4. Drainage tube over the small hole in the center of the adhesive film, connected to 300 mL canister for ACTIV.A.C.TM therapy system and a portable KSI VAC negative pressure wound system pump.

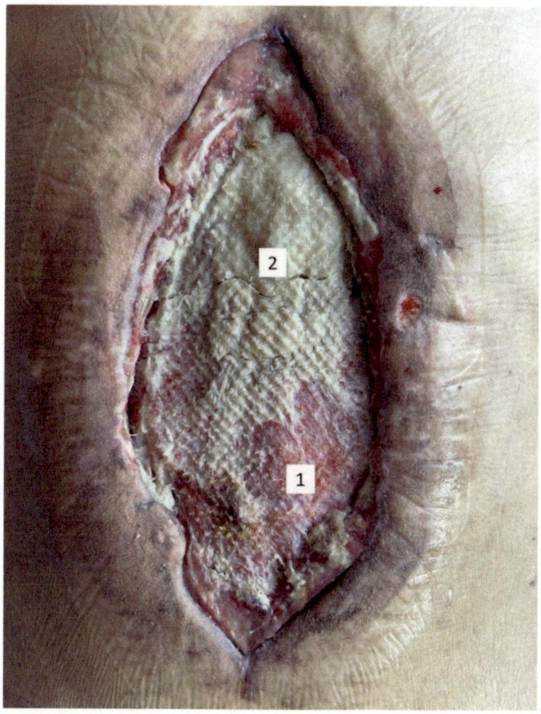

Figure 6.
The 23rd postoperative day after transfascial intraperitoneal placement and fixation of Ovitex® 2S–P reinformed tissue matrix of 25 × 40 cm size for definitive abdominal closure. Digits: 1 – advancing granulation tissue; the shape of the polypropylene grid pattern is visible on the surface of granulations. 2 – partially degrading biological substance of the mesh.

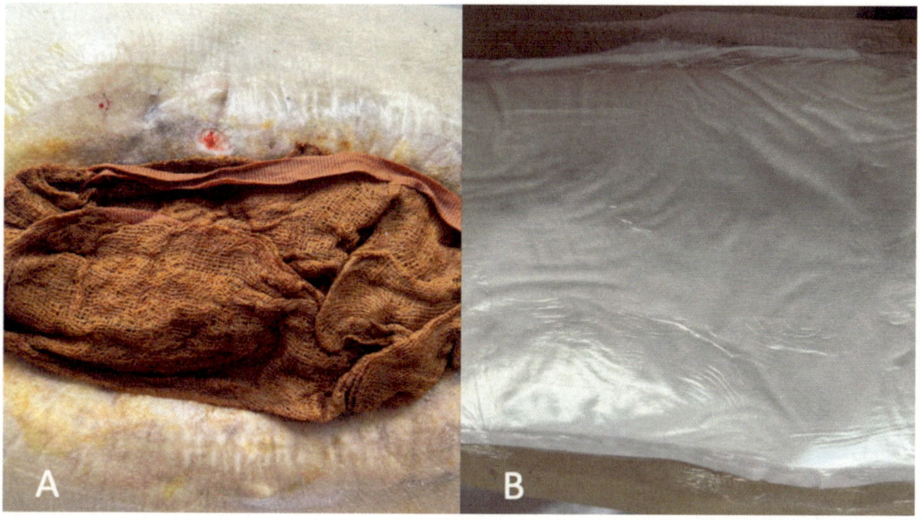

Figure 7.
Post-negative therapy granulating wound care. A: the granulating wound is covered by Raytex roll gauzes soaked in Betadine® solution; of not;, it was changed to Flaminal® Hydro (Enzyme Alginogel) dressings as wound exuding was very mild. B: 3 M Kerramax Care™ super-absorbent dressing of 20 × 30 cm size covers the Raytex roll gauzes; semi-permeable ClearFilms fix the dressing to the skin.

an alternative to prosthetic mesh. The procedure involves four steps: first, developing and dissecting the skin flaps of the anterior abdominal wall out to the anterior superior iliac spine and the chest wall; second, dividing the aponeurosis of the external oblique muscle lateral to the semilunar line, extending to the chest wall at the horizontal level of the xiphoid process; third, freeing the external oblique muscle to enable the rectus myofascial component to be mobilized medially; fourth, restoration of the midline [7].

In general, abdominal component separation techniques—posterior, such as retro-muscular Rives-Stoppa type and transverse abdominis release, or a combination of these two, and anterior—should be considered for elective incisional hernia repair and not used for the management of OA in emergency surgery settings. However, these techniques can be applied in carefully selected lower-risk patients after primary vascular or parenchymal organ trauma surgery [50]. Patient-centered and shared decision-making are two fundamental principles in patient care.

Using mesh during abdominal wall reconstruction significantly reduces the recurrence rate of hernias and is now the preferred repair method. However, mesh placement plays a critical role in the procedure's success as the anatomical position of biological mesh influences recurrence rates. Mesh onlay positioning or bridging with mesh is less favorable and is associated with higher recurrence rates. A meta-analysis showed that component separation with primary fascial closure and mesh reinforcement has a lower risk of hernia recurrence than bridged repairs. When biologic mesh is used to bridge a gap and sewn to the edge of the fascia, recurrence rates can reach as high as 80%. In contrast, when the fascia is reapproximated and the mesh is used to reinforce the repair, the recurrence rate drops to approximately 20% [51].

Although abdominal wall component separation has become the commonly used technique for elective incisional hernia repairs, its effectiveness for definitive closure of an OA still needs to be clarified. In general, its use in acute surgery settings, particularly in the presence of ongoing intra-abdominal sepsis and visceral and abdominal wall edema, is not recommended. However, favorable scenarios in the non-contaminated abdominal cavities and walls are possible [11, 50–52].

7.2.3.1 Scenario, vascular and general surgery settings

A scenario of definitive closure of the abdominal wall using one of the component separation techniques after full evisceration following complex vascular surgery is as follows:

Emergency open transperitoneal aortoiliac aneurysm repair using a bifurcated polyester graft was performed on a patient in the 60s. On postoperative day 9, the patient underwent the second emergency surgery because of the full evisceration of the small intestine and transverse colon. A serosal tear was identified in the middle portion of the transverse colon. No signs of contamination of the peritoneal cavity were observed. AbThera™ with active negative pressure therapy was applied for the temporary closure of the abdomen. On postoperative day 10, the exploratory relaparotomy was performed. OA was classed as 1A. Abdominal wall reconstruction was performed by the retro-muscular (Rives-Stoppa) method, using Ovitex® 1S–P reinformed tissue matrix of 25 × 40 cm size. Sublay negative pressure drainage was activated. Further postoperative period was uneventful. The patient has fully recovered after these three emergency abdominal operations and was discharged from both abdominal wall reconstruction and vascular surgery clinics 5 months later.

7.2.4 Dynamic retention sutures

Section 5 of this chapter, titled "Dynamic retention sutures: an abdominal approximation anchor, ABRA®", describes this technique, which can be used for temporary and definitive abdominal closure. The ABRA® system can achieve delayed abdominal closure within 30 days, with a median application duration of 7 days in 61–88% of cases. However, this system can be painful and uncomfortable for the patients and may result in unsightly scarring and ulcerations, so it is important to apply reasonable tension [33].

7.2.5 The importance of using a combination of methods to close the abdominal wall

No single technique consistently yields optimal results, particularly in patients with peritonitis or traumatic injuries. Individual methods, while beneficial, often have limitations when used in isolation. For example, negative pressure therapy promotes granulation and abdominal fluid management. However, it may not be sufficient to achieve a full fascial closure. Similarly, dynamic suturing and mesh-mediated techniques provide the necessary tension to approximate the fascia. Still, they may be enhanced by the additional benefits of negative pressure therapy in evacuating fluids and reducing the risk of intraabdominal complications. Therefore, combining different methods for abdominal wall closure is crucial for achieving the best clinical outcomes for patients with OA [53].

Negative pressure therapy combined with dynamic components—like mesh-mediated fascial traction or dynamic sutures—has been shown to yield the best delayed fascial closure rates. A systematic review of publications addressing the treatment of the OA in patients with peritonitis of nontraumatic origin found that the highest

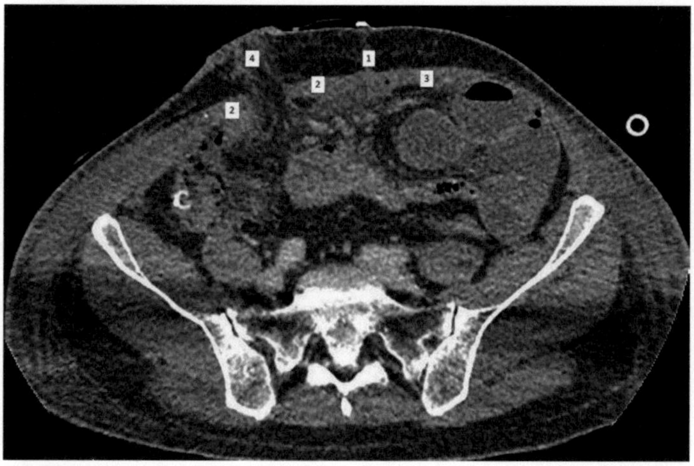

Figure 8.
Anterior abdominal wall radiological anatomy after end ileostomy formation and definitive abdominal wall closure following two damage-control laparotomies with temporary abdominal closure utilizing a 3M™ AbThera™ advanced open abdomen dressing system; all three operations were performed within 72 hours from the moment of the primary emergency surgery. Digits: 1 – linea alba. 2 – right rectus abdominis muscle. 3 – left rectus abdominis muscle. 4 – end ileostomy. Synopsis of the case: Please see the synopsis for ***Figure 1****. After the next 48 hours, a second re-exploration of the abdominal cavity and a standard end ileostomy were performed. The abdominal wall was closed by layers. Linea alba was approximated using two loop-PDS (polydioxanone) size 1 continuous sutures. The skin was closed using metallic clips. The patient survived.*

fascial closure rate was seen for negative pressure wound therapy with fascial traction (73.1%) and dynamic retention sutures (73.6%) [53]. However, careful selection and combination of abdominal wall closure techniques are essential for achieving optimal outcomes in each surgical context, as definitive closure is notably more challenging in OA patients with peritonitis compared to those with traumatic injuries to the parenchymal abdominal organs requiring effective packing and temporary closure of the abdominal wall.

By integrating temporary and definitive abdominal wall closure techniques, surgeons can customize their approach to meet each patient's specific needs, improving survival and abdominal wall closure rates, reducing complications, and enhancing overall clinical outcomes. This multifaceted strategy is particularly crucial in complex surgical environments when the ability to adapt and combine methods can significantly impact the procedure's success. Careful selection and combination of abdominal wall closure techniques are essential for achieving optimal outcomes in each surgical context (**Figure 8**).

8. Incisional hernia as a long-term sequela after definitive abdominal closure

An incisional hernia is a potential long-term sequela that can develop following definitive abdominal closure in any patient. However, various patient, disease, trauma, surgical technique, and postoperative factors influence the risk of developing an incisional hernia—for example, fascial bridging, inadequate fascial reinforcement, postoperative increased intra-abdominal pressure, and abdominal wall tissue ischemia and infection.

Various studies assessed the long-term incidence of incisional hernias following OA. For example, Bjørsum-Meyer's study, which included 14 participants treated with vacuum-assisted wound closure and mesh-mediated fascial traction, detected a 21% rate of incisional hernia confirmed by computed tomography [52]. This rate was observed over a follow-up period ranging from 1 to 36 months, with a median of 21 months.

Petersson et al. studied 11 patients who received vacuum-assisted wound closure combined with permanent onlay mesh–mediated fascial traction. The study reported a 100% success rate in fascial closure and no mortality within 30 days. Among the nine patients eligible for incisional hernia follow-up (with a median of 467 days, which is 15.6 months), two (22.2%) patients developed hernias [54].

In the study by Brandl et al., which involved 112 patients, 35% of those who underwent vacuum-assisted delayed primary fascia closure with dynamic vessel loops developed incisional hernias. This finding was observed over a median follow-up period of 26 months, ranging from 12 to 81 months [55].

These three selected studies demonstrate that incisional hernia is a common adverse medical effect—21, 22, and 35%—even after applying the combination of best methods to close the abdominal wall. They also show that an incisional hernia can occur at any time—weeks, months, or even years after the definitive abdominal wall surgery—and that incisional hernia occurrence increases over time. The medians of the follow-up period were less than 2 years in the first two studies and more than 2 years in the third study [52, 54, 55].

It is important to follow evidence-based practice and use the best abdominal wall closure methods to minimize postoperative morbidity in patients to whom OA was a

DOI: http://dx.doi.org/10.5772/intechopen.1008568

necessary treatment option at the point of intraabdominal catastrophe. Even efficient management of chronic cough, malnutrition, overweight, or obesity can help reduce the likelihood of hernia disease development.

9. Conclusions

Primary goals in open abdomen management: When treating patients with an OA, the surgeon's foremost objectives are to preserve the patient's life; reduce disease, trauma, and surgery-related morbidity; and achieve abdominal closure. The latter objective involves either securing primary fascial closure or bridging the fascial gap if primary closure is impossible within 1 week or, in exceptional cases, within 8–10 days.

Strategy for initial closure attempts: If a primary fascial repair cannot be achieved during the initial laparotomy, the best approach is temporarily covering the abdomen using negative pressure systems. This— provided the patient's physiological condition is satisfactory or good—should be supplemented with synthetic mesh-mediated traction to approximate the fascial edges when it is anatomically possible. Targeted packing of the abdominal wall is indicated in selected trauma and some non-trauma emergency patients.

Alternative closure methods: If direct suturing of the fascia remains unfeasible after 2–3 surgical attempts of mesh-mediated traction, the fascial gap should be bridged using purely biological or polypropylene-reinforced biological meshes with a non-cross-linked collagenic structure. However, fascial bridging as a definitive abdominal closure method should be considered early if a robust clinical prediction is that 2–3 surgical attempts of mesh-mediated traction will fail.

When bridging is not possible: If bridging the fascial gap is impossible, the abdomen should be covered solely with skin. This can be achieved through primary closure with subcutaneous flaps, applying a skin graft, or other advanced plastic surgery techniques.

Abdominal wall reconstruction: For cases where primary fascial closure is unachievable, abdominal wall reconstructions—such as retro-rectus (preferred) or anterior component separation (the alternative for some cases)—can be considered, provided there are no signs of abdominal contamination or infection in physiologically stable patients.

Managing incisional hernia: Incisional hernia is common following definitive abdominal wall closure, reaching up to 80% in fascial gap-bridging surgery. Patients should be informed about this potential outcome and provided with appropriate counseling.

Timing for elective abdominal wall reconstruction in patients with computed tomography-proven incisional hernia: Surgery is recommended 12 months after achieving complete primary abdominal wall closure or after healing by secondary intention.

Multidisciplinary approach: Effective management of OA and its potential sequelae requires a multidisciplinary approach throughout the patient's hospital stay and post-discharge period. Follow-up is the key.

Author details

Svetlana Doris Brincat[1*] and Raimundas Lunevicius[2]

1 Department of Surgery, Mater Dei Hospital, Msida, Malta

2 Department of General Surgery, Liverpool University Hospitals NHS Foundation Trust, Liverpool, UK

*Address all correspondence to: svetlana-doris.brincat@gov.mt

References

[1] José Santivañez Palominos J, Arturo V, Manuel C. Open abdomen: The surgeons' challenge. In: Dogan KH, editor. Wound Healing - Current Perspectives. London, UK: IntechOpen; 2019. DOI: 10.5772/intechopen.81428

[2] Beckman M, Paul J, Neideen T, Weigelt JA. Role of the open abdomen in critically ill patients. Critical Care Clinics. 2016;**32**:255-264. DOI: 10.1016/j.ccc.2015.12.003

[3] Roberts DJ, Leppäniemi A, Tolonen M, Mentula P, Björck M, Kirkpatrick AW, et al. The open abdomen in trauma, acute care, and vascular and endovascular surgery: Comprehensive, expert, narrative review. BJS Open. 2023;7:84. DOI: 10.1093/bjsopen/zrad084

[4] Leguit P. Zip-closure of the abdomen. The Netherlands Journal of Surgery. 1982;**34**:40-41

[5] Feliciano DV, Borraez Gaona OA. Origin of the Bogota bag and its application. In: Duchesne J, Inaba K, Khan AK, editors. Damage Control in Trauma Care. USA: Springer Cham; 2018. pp. 1-7. DOI: 10.1007/978-3-319-72607-6_1

[6] Kron IL, Harman PK, Nolan SP. The measurement of intra-abdominal pressure as a criterion for abdominal re-exploration. Annals of Surgery. 1984;**199**:28-30. DOI: 10.1097/00000658-198401000-00005

[7] Ramirez OM, Ruas E, Dellon AL. "Components separation" method for closure of abdominal-wall defects: An anatomic and clinical study. Plastic and Reconstructive Surgery. 1990;**86**:519-526. DOI: 10.1097/00006534-199009000-00023

[8] Wittmann DH, Aprahamian C, Bergstein JM. Etappenlavage: Advanced diffuse peritonitis managed by planned multiple laparotomies utilizing zippers, slide fastener, and Velcro analogue for temporary abdominal closure. World Journal of Surgery. 1990;**14**:218-226. DOI: 10.1007/BF01664876

[9] Schein M. Planned reoperations and open management in critical intra-abdominal infections: Prospective experience in 52 cases. World Journal of Surgery. 1991;**15**:537-545. DOI: 10.1007/BF01675658

[10] Brock WB, Barker DE, Burns RP. Temporary closure of open abdominal wounds: The vacuum pack. The American Surgeon. 1995;**61**:30-35

[11] Argenta LC, Morykwas MJ. Vacuum-assisted closure: A new method for wound control and treatment: Clinical experience. Annals of Plastic Surgery. 1997;**38**:563-576

[12] Garner GB, Ware DN, Cocanour CS, Duke JH, McKinley BA, Kozar RA, et al. Vacuum-assisted wound closure provides early fascial reapproximation in trauma patients with open abdomens. American Journal of Surgery. 2001;**182**:630-638. DOI: 10.1016/s0002-9610(01)00786-3

[13] Miller PR, Thompson JT, Faler BJ, Meredith JW, Chang MC. Late fascial closure in lieu of ventral hernia: The next step in open abdomen management. The Journal of Trauma. 2002;**53**:843-849. DOI: 10.1097/00005373-200211000-00007

[14] Reimer MW, Yelle J-D, Reitsma B, Doumit G, Allen MA, Bell MS. Management of open abdominal wounds with a dynamic fascial closure

system. Canadian Journal of Surgery. 2008;**51**:209-214

[15] Björck M, Bruhin A, Cheatham M, Hinck D, Kaplan M, Manca G, et al. Classification-important step to improve management of patients with an open abdomen. World Journal of Surgery. 2009;**33**:1154-1157. DOI: 10.1007/s00268-009-9996-3

[16] Rezende-Neto J, Rice T, Abreu ES, Rotstein O, Rizoli S. Anatomical, physiological, and logistical indications for the open abdomen: A proposal for a new classification system. World Journal of Emergency Surgery: WJES. 2016;**11**:28. DOI: 10.1186/s13017-016-0083-4

[17] Coccolini F, Roberts D, Ansaloni L, Ivatury R, Gamberini E, Kluger Y, et al. The open abdomen in trauma and non-trauma patients: WSES guidelines. World Journal of Emergency Surgery: WJES. 2018;**13**:7. DOI: 10.1186/s13017-018-0167-4

[18] Baethge C, Goldbeck-Wood S, Mertens S. SANRA-a scale for the quality assessment of narrative review articles. Research Integrity and Peer Review. 2019;**4**:5. DOI: 10.1186/s41073-019-0064-8

[19] Klein Y. Closure of the open abdomen: A practical approach. Current Trauma Reports. 2016;**2**:196-201. DOI: 10.1007/s40719-016-0063-x

[20] Milne DM, Rambhajan A, Ramsingh J, Cawich SO, Naraynsingh V. Managing the open abdomen in damage control surgery: Should skin-only closure be abandoned? Cureus. 2021;**13**:e15489. DOI: 10.7759/cureus.15489

[21] Björck M, Kirkpatrick AW, Cheatham M, Kaplan M, Leppäniemi A, De Waele JJ. Amended classification of the open abdomen. Scandinavian Journal of Surgery. 2016;**105**:5-10. DOI: 10.1177/1457496916631853

[22] Pepe G, Chiarello MM, Bianchi V, Fico V, Altieri G, Tedesco S, et al. Entero-cutaneous and entero-atmospheric fistulas: Insights into management using negative pressure wound therapy. Journal of Clinical Medicine. 2024;**13**:1279. DOI: 10.3390/jcm13051279

[23] Regner JL, Kobayashi L, Coimbra R. Surgical strategies for management of the open abdomen. World Journal of Surgery. 2012;**36**:497-510. DOI: 10.1007/s00268-011-1203-7

[24] The Pediatric Guidelines Sub-Committee for the World Society of the Abdominal Compartment Syndrome, Kirkpatrick AW, Roberts DJ, De Waele J, Jaeschke R, Malbrain MLNG, et al. Intra-abdominal hypertension and the abdominal compartment syndrome: Updated consensus definitions and clinical practice guidelines from the world society of the abdominal compartment syndrome. Intensive Care Medicine. 2013;**39**:1190-1206. DOI: 10.1007/s00134-013-2906-z

[25] Huang Q, Li J, Lau W-Y. Techniques for abdominal wall closure after damage control laparotomy: From temporary abdominal closure to early/delayed fascial closure-a review. Gastroenterology Research and Practice. 2016;**2016**:2073260. DOI: 10.1155/2016/2073260

[26] Heo Y, Kim DH. The temporary abdominal closure techniques used for trauma patients: A systematic review and meta-analysis. Annals of Surgical Treatment and Research. 2023;**104**:237-247. DOI: 10.4174/astr.2023.104.4.237

[27] Latifi R, Higa G, Tilley E. A difficult abdomen: Temporary closure and

management of the consequences. In: Latifi R, editor. Surgery of Complex Abdominal Wall Defects. 2nd ed. Switzerland: Springer Cham; 2017. pp. 77-86. DOI: 10.1007/978-3-319-55868-4_8

[28] Boukerrouche A. Open abdomen and temporarily abdominal closure. Journal of Emergency Medicine Trauma & Surgical Care. 2019;**6**:1-7. DOI: 10.24966/ETS-8798/100034

[29] Brown LR, Rentea RM. Temporary abdominal closure techniques. Treasure Island: StatPearls Publishing [Internet]; 2024. Available from: https://www.ncbi.nlm.nih.gov/books/NBK564378/

[30] Manterola C, Moraga J, Urrutia S. Laparostomía contenida con bolsa de Bogotá. Resultados de una serie de casos [contained laparostomy with a Bogota bag. Results of case series]. Cirugía Española. 2011;**89**:379-385. DOI: 10.1016/j.ciresp.2011.01.010

[31] Cordoba DAL, Cardenas SMF, Bravo OOL, Castro CAT, Anguila JJM, Castro JPM, et al. Bogotá Bag as a conservative measure for open abdomen secondary to intra-abdominal sepsis. Journal of Medical Research and Health Sciences. 2022;**5**(4):1886-1893. DOI: 10.52845/JMRHS/2022-5-4-5

[32] Patel NY, Cogbill TH, Kallies KJ, Mathiason MA. Temporary abdominal closure: Long-term outcomes. The Journal of Trauma. 2011;**70**:769-774. DOI: 10.1097/TA.0b013e318212785e

[33] Montori G, Coccolini F, Tomasoni M, Fugazzola P, Ceresoli M, Catena F, et al. The management of the open abdomen: The temporary closure systems. In: Coccolini F, Ivatury R, Sugrue M, Ansaloni L, editors. Open Abdomen. Hot Topics in Acute Care Surgery and Trauma. USA: Springer Cham; 2018. pp. 119-133. DOI: 10.1186/s13017-018-0167-4

[34] Utiyama EM, Pflug ARM, Damous SHB, Rodrigues AC Jr, de Montero EFS, CAV B. Temporary abdominal closure with zipper-mesh device for management of intra-abdominal sepsis. Revista do Colégio Brasileiro de Cirurgiões. 2015;**42**:18-24. DOI: 10.1590/0100-69912015001005

[35] Perez A, Hilvano S. Abdominal zippers for temporary abdominal closure in planned relaparotomies for peripancreatic sepsis: Experience in a developing country. Journal of Hepato-Biliary-Pancreatic Surgery. 2001;**8**:449-452. DOI: 10.1007/pl00009959

[36] Anastasiu M, Şurlin V, Beuran M. The management of the open abdomen - A literature review. Chirurgia. 2021;**116**(6):645. DOI: 10.21614/chirurgia.116.6.645

[37] Turza KC, Campbell CA, Rosenberger LH, Politano AD, Davies SW, Riccio LM, et al. Options for closure of the infected abdomen. Surgical Infections. 2012;**13**(6):343-351. DOI: 10.1089/sur.2012.014

[38] Fansler RF, Taheri P, Cullinane C, Sabates B, Flint LM. Polypropylene mesh closure of the complicated abdominal wound. American Journal of Surgery. 1995;**170**:15-18. DOI: 10.1016/s0002-9610(99)80244-x

[39] Badylak SF, Gilbert TW. Immune response to biologic scaffold materials. Seminars in Immunology. 2008;**20**:109-116. DOI: 10.1016/j.smim.2007.11.003

[40] Kumar A, FitzGerald J. Biologic versus synthetic mesh reinforcement: What are the pros and cons? Clinics in Colon and Rectal Surgery. 2014;**27**:140-148. DOI: 10.1055/s-0034-1394155

[41] Barker DE, Green JM, Maxwell RA, Smith PW, Mejia VA, Dart BW, et al.

Experience with vacuum-pack temporary abdominal wound closure in 258 trauma and general and vascular surgical patients. Journal of the American College of Surgeons. 2007;**204**:784-792. DOI: 10.1016/j.jamcollsurg.2006.12.039

[42] 3M Company. 3MTM AbThera™ Open Abdomen Negative Pressure Therapy [Internet]. 2021. Available from: https://multimedia.3m.com/mws/media/2139348O/3m-abthera-openabdomen-negative-pressure-therapyproduct-monograph-us.pdf [Accessed: October 13, 2024]

[43] Cheatham ML, Demetriades D, Fabian TC, Kaplan MJ, Miles WS, Schreiber MA, et al. Prospective study examining clinical outcomes associated with a negative pressure wound therapy system and Barker's vacuum packing technique. World Journal of Surgery. 2013;**37**:2018-2030. DOI: 10.1007/s00268-013-2080-z

[44] Kirkpatrick AW, Roberts DJ, Faris PD, Ball CG, Kubes P, Tiruta C, et al. Active negative pressure peritoneal therapy after abbreviated laparotomy: The intraperitoneal vacuum randomized controlled trial. Annals of Surgery. 2015;**262**:38-46. DOI: 10.1097/SLA.0000000000001095

[45] Lammers D, Conner J, Rokayak O, Rakestraw S, Hardin RD, Gillis SC, et al. Management strategies for the open abdomen following damage control laparotomy. Current Trauma Reports. 2023;**9**:140-148. DOI: 10.1007/s40719-023-00262-8

[46] Deerenberg EB, Henriksen NA, Antoniou GA, Antoniou SA, Bramer WM, Fischer JP, et al. Updated guideline for closure of abdominal wall incisions from the European and American hernia societies. The British Journal of Surgery. 2022;**109**:1239-1250. DOI: 10.1093/bjs/znac302

[47] Fasciotens. Abdominal wall solutions [Internet]. 2024. Available from: https://www.fasciotens.com/ [Accessed: October 13, 2024]

[48] Fung S, Ashmawy H, Krieglstein C, Halama T, Schilawa D, Fuckert O, et al. Vertical traction device prevents abdominal wall retraction and facilitates early primary fascial closure of septic and non-septic open abdomen. Langenbeck's Archives of Surgery. 2022;**407**:2075-2083. DOI: 10.1007/s00423-021-02424-1

[49] National Institute for Health and Care Excellence. Fasciotens for Abdominal Wall Closure [Internet]. 2023. Available from: www.nice.org.uk/guidance/mib321 [Accessed: October 13, 2024]

[50] York and Scarborough Teaching Hospital. Complex abdominal wall hernia. [Internet]. 2022. Available from: https://www.yorkhospitals.nhs.uk/seecmsfile/?id=2943 [Accessed: October 13, 2024]

[51] Köckerling F, Alam NN, Antoniou SA, Daniels IR, Famiglietti F, Fortelny RH, et al. What is the evidence for the use of biologic or biosynthetic meshes in abdominal wall reconstruction? Hernia. 2018;**22**:249-269. DOI: 10.1007/s10029-018-1735-y

[52] Bjørsum-Meyer T, Skarbye M, Jensen KH. Vacuum with mesh is a feasible temporary closure device after fascial dehiscence. Danish Medical Journal. 2013;**60**:A4719

[53] Atema JJ, Gans SL, Boermeester MA. Systematic review and meta-analysis of the open abdomen and temporary abdominal closure techniques in non-trauma patients. World Journal of Surgery. 2015;**39**:912-925. DOI: 10.1007/s00268-014-2883-6

[54] Petersson P, Montgomery A, Petersson U. Vacuum-assisted wound

closure and permanent onlay mesh-mediated fascial traction: A novel technique for the prevention of incisional hernia after open abdomen therapy including results from a retrospective case series. Scandinavian Journal of Surgery. 2019;**108**:216-226. DOI: 10.1177/1457496918818979

[55] Brandl A, Laimer E, Perathoner A, Zitt M, Pratschke J, Kafka-Ritsch R. Incisional hernia rate after open abdomen treatment with negative pressure and delayed primary fascia closure. Hernia. 2014;**18**:105-111. DOI: 10.1007/s10029-013-1064-0